VALITEQ ™

ASEPTIC TECHNIQUE VALIDATION SYSTEM

COMPOUNDING MANUAL

MARGHI R. McKEON
GREGORY F. PETERS

SECOND EDITION

EDITOR
JAMES C. BOYLAN

ADVISORY PANEL
JAMES C. BOYLAN, R.Ph., Ph.D.
KATHARINE L. KOSHEL, Pharm.D.
SUSAN M. TEDESCO, CPhT
SALVATORE J. TURCO, Pharm.D., FASHP

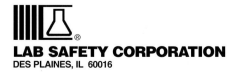

LAB SAFETY CORPORATION
DES PLAINES, IL 60016

Lab Safety Corporation
1245 Rand Road, Des Plaines, IL 60016
tel: 877-699-7304; fax: 847-699-7040

ISBN: 0-9708302-3-8

Current printing (last digit):
10 9 8 7 6 5 4 3 2

PREFACE

Human use of medicinal plants to combat disease, pain, and parasitic infestation predates civilization. Agriculture originated when medicine men began cultivating important drug plants, then broadened to include the food crops which enabled humans to abandon their hunting and gathering lifestyles. However, until recently, the only routes of drug administration available to physicians were inhalation, ingestion, and topical absorption.

The advent of intravenous (IV) administration of drugs was an important advance in medicine. It improved the efficacy of many products that were poorly absorbed or destroyed by the digestive system, and allowed for the use of better-controlled doses of potent substances. In addition, IV therapy distributes the drug throughout the body within seconds, speeding the nutritional, pain-relieving, and disease-fighting processes.

There are, however, potential drawbacks to IV therapy. It is a form of parenteral route administration which bypasses most of the body's natural defense systems, and can spread harmful substances as quickly and widely as it does useful drugs. The introduction of infectious agents and other foreign materials directly into the bloodstream can be harmful or fatal to the patient.

Manufacturers of drug products are subject to strict rules, known as the Current Good Manufacturing Practices (cGMPs)[1], and must incorporate a validated scientific basis of ensuring that drug products are pure, sterile, non-pyrogenic, and free of any particulates or breakdown products. Manufacturers of tubing, IV bags, bottles, syringes and other medical devices must meet similar criteria. The packaging of drugs and equipment is designed to preserve product integrity and sterility through shipment and storage. When pharmacy personnel open this packaging to compound patient doses, they create the opportunity for contamination or adulteration of the product.

While the cGMPs are not applicable to Pharmacy operations, it is in the interest of the patient population and the profession of Pharmacy as a whole to institute standardized quality assurance measures which assure the safety of all medications produced by the Pharmacy. The VALITEQ™ Aseptic Technique Validation System is an essential step in assuring the achievement of this goal.

ACKNOWLEDGMENTS

The authors wish to thank the following individuals and client institutions for their contributions and tireless support of the Lab Safety Corporation Validation and Monitoring System for IV Admixtures, from which the VALITEQ™ Aseptic Technique Validation System is derived.

Marianne Chan, Pharm.D.
Director of Pharmacy Services
The Children's Memorial Hospital
Chicago, Illinois

Jerome Ochab, R.Ph., M.B.A.
Director of Pharmacy
Ravenswood Hospital Medical Center
Chicago, Illinois

Debra M. Tennant, Pharm.D.
Pharmacy Manager
Highland Park Hospital
Highland Park, Illinois

CONTENTS

PART THREE: BARRIER CONTROLS

PART FOUR: ASEPTIC MANIPULATIONS

EDUCATIONAL GOAL

The goal of this course is to educate supervisory and technical personnel involved in the IV compounding process in both the theory and practices that assure the safety and efficacy of the IV products they compound and dispense.

USE OF THIS MANUAL

This compounding manual is divided into five sections:

I. **QUALITY ASSURANCE THEORY FOR IV ADMIXTURES**

II. **ENGINEERING CONTROLS AND LAMINAR AIRFLOW THEORY**

III. **BARRIER CONTROLS**

IV. **ASEPTIC MANIPULATIONS**

V. **PHARMACEUTICAL COMPOUNDING CALCULATIONS**

The concepts and methods presented in this manual should be studied and practiced carefully. Several study techniques that may be helpful to you have been incorporated. We suggest you try some of these techniques as you read.

Learning Objectives: Learning objectives are defined at the beginning of each section. The text in each section is subdivided by learning objective, and a fundamental **"Key Concept"** supporting each learning objective is then presented, followed by discussion of additional details and practical applications. As you read the text, refer often to both the learning objective, and the key concept to see how these points relate to the learning objective. **Think of ways the topic being discussed relates to your own work situation.**

Definitions: Important terms and definitions are presented at the beginning of each section. Unless you are certain that you understand each term completely ***as it applies to IV compounding***, refer back to the definition when you encounter the term in the discussion. Be sure you understand all terms and definitions; you will encounter them frequently throughout this course.

Self-evaluation: A written self-evaluation is provided at the end of each section. The page on which the topic of the question is discussed is listed following each question, and the self-evaluation answers are provided at the end of the manual. As you finish each section, please complete the self-evaluation exercise without referring to the text or answers (write your answers on a separate piece of paper). Check your answers and review the portion of text relating to any questions you missed. Be sure you understand **why** your answer was incorrect. When you have completed the manual, again complete the self-evaluations. Any questions missed twice should alert you to potential problem areas, which may require additional study or assistance.

Training Video Series: Although this manual can be used as a "stand-alone" course, many concepts are more easily understood when they are presented visually. The VALITEQ™ Training Video series, presented on three VHS cassettes, parallels the material in this manual and illustrates many concepts and techniques that are difficult to describe through the written word alone. Viewing this series may clarify certain concepts and help you to imprint them into your visual memory more effectively. **However, this manual contains important information which is not presented in the video.**

Group Discussion: Because IV admixtures compounding is a cooperative activity, it is usually useful to discuss the concepts presented in this course with your co-workers, paying particular attention to the issues that relate to your institution's unique applications. The emphasis in all such discussions should be constructive, rather than critical.

Guided Practice: The ultimate goal of this course is to improve your IV compounding skills. Transferring knowledge to actual daily work routines requires practice. It is recommended that all personnel have their pharmacy Preceptor or other qualified "coach" observe them while they are learning each technique, because it is important that you perform the techniques correctly when you practice. You may also find that taking a turn as the observer helps you become more aware of the many small errors that can be made while compounding.

WRITTEN AND PRACTICAL SKILLS ASSESSMENTS

Written and practical assessments will cover all information presented in this manual, and information provided in the VALITEQ™ Training Video series. Practical assessment criteria are presented at the end of the manual.

I. QUALITY ASSURANCE THEORY FOR IV ADMIXTURES

LEARNING OBJECTIVES FOR SECTION I.

Upon completion of this section you should be able to:

Objective 1.1) Understand the need for the application of aseptic processing in IV compounding, and define potential hazards to the patient associated with IV therapy.

Objective 1.2) Understand the rationale supporting Quality Assurance release of sterile IV admixtures, and describe the differences between Quality Assurance (QA) and Quality Control (QC) as they relate to control of variables in IV compounding programs.

Objective 1.3) Understand and explain the role of engineering controls, barrier controls, and personnel disciplines in the production of unadulterated IV admixtures.

Objective 1.4) Understand and explain the role of both the individual and the team in the production of acceptable-quality IV products.

TERMS FOR SECTION I.

Aseptic Processing	A system of operations designed and validated to prevent the introduction of pathogenic microorganisms, which may lead to sepsis (a state of infection or disease).
Contaminant	Any impurity.
Cross-contamination	Contamination of one drug with another.
Engineering Controls	Equipment and mechanical systems designed to achieve control of specific environmental conditions, including levels of airborne particulates, microorganisms, temperature, humidity, lighting, and noise.
Monitoring	A system of ongoing verifications demonstrating that the conditions validated to achieve acceptable product quality continue in effect over time.

Parenteral	Administration of drugs by a route other than through the digestive tract.
Pathogenic	Disease-causing.
Pyrogenic	Literally "fire-causing"; substances which cause fever or inflamation. Pyrogens are endotoxins, usually residues or fragments of decomposed microorganisms.
Quality Assurance	A system assuring that a product meets specified quality criteria by demonstrating its production in compliance with a properly validated and monitored process, under defined conditions.
Quality Control	A system ensuring that a product meets specified criteria by successful testing prior to product release.
Validation	A system of proofs demonstrating that a process operates adequately to achieve the defined product quality levels, and that personnel have the required skills to repeatedly perform the defined process.
Variable	Any factor having a range of possible values which may affect product quality. The goal of process design is to control variables in ways that optimize product quality.

Objective 1.1) Understand the need for the application of aseptic processing in IV compounding, and define potential hazards to the patient associated with IV therapy.

Key Concept: Natural routes for absorption of drugs include the gut, lungs, skin, and other vascularized epithelia which provide a barrier to many harmful contaminants. Because drugs introduced directly into the bloodstream bypass the body's normal systems of defense against invasion by microorganisms and other foreign materials, methods must be used to keep these products free of materials that may cause harm to the patient. The goal of aseptic processing is to assure that all pharmacy-prepared IV drug products are free of all contaminants. Contaminants of concern include:

1) **Particulate Matter,**
2) **Microorganisms,**
3) **Allergens,**
4) **Pyrogens, and**
5) **Drug Residues.**

PARTICULATE MATTER

Microscopic fragments of glass, dust, rubber, plastic, fibers and other debris may cause occlusion of the peripheral vasculature in any part of the body, such as the brain, eyes, or lungs, resulting in a variety of adverse effects. Improper cleaning, sanitizing, and manipulative technique may lead to the introduction of foreign matter into IV solutions. "Cores" of stopper material from vial septa, fragments of glass produced when ampules are opened, skin debris, lint, and dust are common sources of particulate contamination[2]. Precipitation of drug product due to incompatibility of additives, improper mixing, or inappropriate solution concentration may also produce particulates, and lead to incorrect dosage.

MICROORGANISMS

Pathogenic (disease-causing) microorganisms generally include viruses, bacteria, fungi, and parasites, which are known as **pathogens.** Intravenous introduction of microorganisms can lead to serious sepsis or disease, because many, normally non-pathogenic microorganisms may become pathogenic when introduced directly into the bloodstream. Nature seeks biodiversity, and will take advantage of any opportunity to invade and infect the body. Potential sources of microbial contamination are numerous.

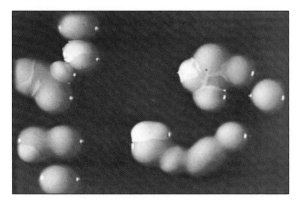

Bacteria and fungi may be introduced into IV preparations through the **air,** through **water** and other liquids, or from **surface contamination** on work surfaces, vials, bags, wrappers and supplies. The most common route of contamination of IV admixtures is surface contamination by **touch.**

ALLERGENS

Many foreign substances, such as molds, pollen, dust, and various proteins can produce an allergic response in sensitive individuals. A growing number of patients and practitioners are exhibiting allergic reactions to latex. Latex is a common component of gloves, tubing, and vial and admixture port closure systems. Although

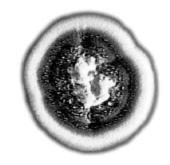

latex-free gloves are becoming more commonly used, and vial closures and tubing are becoming increasingly available in latex-free forms, care should be exercised to avoid introducing latex glove powder into admixtures. This may occur if glove powder is allowed to contaminate the critical work zone.

PYROGENS

Many non-viable substances, if introduced into the bloodstream, may result in a **pyrogenic (fever-causing; inflammatory)** response that may cause serious harm to the patient. Pyrogenic agents may include **non-biological particulates,** as well as cell wall fragments, and other residues of microorganisms, which have been killed **(endotoxins)**. Pyrogens may enter solutions by the same routes as pathogens.

Remember, patients are ill and may be incapable of resisting infections and inflammations, placing them at greater risk than healthy individuals.

DRUG RESIDUES

IV solutions should be free of cross-contamination by drugs used in previous compounding procedures which may be harmful to a patient for whom they are not intended, or which may produce an adverse drug interaction or allergy. Alcohol can also be a contaminant of this type. To avoid cross-contamination, frequent and thorough cleaning of the work space is critical, especially between batches. This is a component of **line clearance,** which should include removal of all labels and materials not related to the compounding task at hand, and cleaning and sanitizing of the critical work zone. The presence of old labels, left-over additives, used compounding devices, and drug residues may lead to cross-contamination and other errors. Syringes must not be reused for different drugs. Careful reading of labels is also critical to assure that the patient receives the proper medication.

Objective 1.2) Understand the rationale supporting Quality Assurance release of sterile IV admixtures, and describe the differences between Quality Assurance (QA) and Quality Control (QC) as they relate to control of variables in IV compounding programs.

Key Concept: IV products are prepared immediately prior to use and often have limited stability. Therefore, they cannot be tested for sterility, apyrogenicity, potency, and purity prior to use. In a manufacturing setting, testing is performed before a batch of product is released to prove that it meets all criteria[3]. This type of pre-release testing system is known as **Quality Control (QC)**. When QC measures cannot be employed due to time constraints, a **Quality Assurance (QA)** approach must be used to assure that product is of acceptable quality. In order to justify product release using a QA system, the following conditions must be demonstrated.

The *environmental conditions* under which the product is produced must be defined and controlled to minimize the introduction of contaminants from the environment and personnel. Environmental control is also necessary to optimize the compounding environment, and to eliminate the possibility of uncontrolled variables such as environmental particulate levels, temperature, relative humidity, poor lighting levels, operator hygiene, etc., adversely effecting product. Engineering controls, cleaning, gowning, materials staging, housekeeping, and maintenance procedures are employed to assure that the compounding environment meets pre-established criteria.

The *process* used must be capable of consistently producing admixtures of acceptable quality. It must be carefully examined to identify possible routes of contamination. **An exact method for performing each process step in a way that eliminates contamination potential is then developed, challenged, and established in written policies and procedures.** Strict and consistent adherence to these procedures is essential. Procedures must be reviewed whenever new equipment or products are introduced, and periodically, to assure their continued relevance and efficacy.

The *personnel* must be capable of consistently performing processing activities to produce admixtures of acceptable quality. **Personnel are the key component of any system.** Appropriate qualifications should be established and detailed written job descriptions provided to all staff members. Policies and procedures must be written and communicated through an effective training program, with regular, periodic reassessment of knowledge and skills.

Quality Assurance protocols employ a **"validation and monitoring"** approach to demonstrate that these essential, pre-defined conditions are met. Initially, validation of the process and personnel competency in the controlled work environment is accomplished by performing a **"media-fill validation"**. The intended process is performed using a sterile growth medium in place of actual product. This medium is highly susceptible to contamination resulting from any breach in process control. If no growth in these representative media-filled products occurs, it may then be assumed that no viable contaminants have been introduced by the compounding procedure under the environmental conditions that existed at the time of the test. The validation process should be repeated in triplicate for minimum statistical reasons, in order to demonstrate consistency[4].

Following validation, **ongoing monitoring** of the production system, and documentation of specific tasks (such as cleaning), are employed to **verify that production is being carried out under the validated conditions, using the validated process.** Monitoring may include periodic tests of engineering controls and environmental cleanliness, personnel testing, verification of vial content and plunger positions, and other factors which may compromise product quality. End-product sterility testing should also be included in monitoring activities. In a QA scenario, however, end-product testing is not a pre-release method of proving product sterility (a product parameter). It is, rather a *"spot-check"* to verify that the **process** is operating within **acceptable quality limits** (a process parameter). *When variables are outside the validated range, it is impossible to reliably predict product quality.*

Because documentation of task completion and monitoring of process parameters are the sole methods available to demonstrate product acceptability prior to release, personnel must follow and document all procedures in strict accordance with established policies. The rule is:

"If you didn't write it down, you didn't do it!"

Objective 1.3) Understand and explain the role of engineering controls, barrier controls, and personnel disciplines in the production of unadulterated IV admixtures.

Key Concept: A method of compounding must be employed that is demonstrated to be effective in preventing contamination of IV solutions. This method, generally referred to as aseptic processing, incorporates several different strategies into an integrated, overlapping system to prevent contamination. The three main strategies of an aseptic processing system are:

> *Engineering controls:* **Equipment** designed to provide a renewable, aseptic, controlled environment in which to work, limiting **contamination potential,**

> *Barrier controls:* **Physical barriers** which reduce the transmission of contaminants to the product, limiting **contamination transfer,** and

> *Personnel controls (Aseptic technique):* **Manipulative methods** which reduce transmission of contaminants to the product, limiting **contamination events.**

None of these components **alone** provides complete product protection, all of the time. An effective aseptic processing system provides redundancy to reduce the risk of contamination in the event that any single device or technique fails, or is defeated. Unfortunately, it is usually impossible for pharmacy to detect the failure of a technique or device, because no prerelease testing is performed. To effectively prevent adulteration of drug products, compounding personnel must understand and properly employ each component of the aseptic processing system.

Laminar Airflow **(LAF)** Workstations **(hoods)**, as primary engineering controls, will be discussed in detail in Section II. Each type of LAF hood provides specific benefits, but also has limitations. It is essential that all personnel understand the equipment they rely upon when performing their compounding duties.

Barrier use is an aid to aseptic technique and is discussed in Section III. Institutional policies vary on some specific barrier use, however, it is recommended that full gowning be employed as described. Additional care in manipulative technique must be exercised if barrier items are omitted from your institutional gowning requirements.

Regardless of the engineering and barrier controls employed to limit contamination potential, it is the manipulative technique of personnel that will ultimately support or defeat these controls, leading to contamination events. Aseptic technique is discussed in Section IV.

Objective 1.4) Understand and explain the role of both the individual and the team in the production of acceptable-quality IV products.

Key Concept: The quality of a product is determined at the time of compounding by the person who performs the compounding. A team approach to the IV admixtures process is necessary to support individuals performing compounding duties to assure the highest level of confidence in the IV product.

Quality Assurance validation and monitoring, combined with engineering controls, barrier controls, and training in manipulative techniques, provide a system and environment to support the key component of the IV admixtures compounding program, namely, compounding personnel. The identity, concentration, and purity of compounded IV products is determined at the time of compounding, by the individual performing the manipulations. No amount of care and testing by manufacturers, laminar airflow equipment, cleanrooms or gowning can reverse errors in dosage or technique on the part of compounding personnel. This places tremendous responsibility on the individual, who may perform hundreds of aseptic manipulations daily.

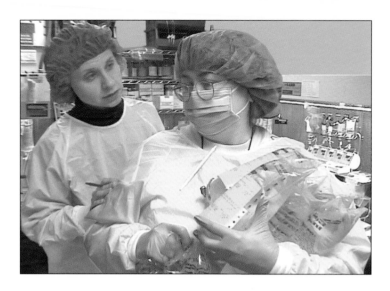

No human, or for that matter, no machine, can function perfectly all of the time. The individual performing compounding requires a **team** of supporting personnel. Housekeeping, maintenance and engineering staff play important roles in maintaining the quality of the compounding environment. These support personnel require special training to perform their duties properly, and all procedures performed by these personnel should be documented. Purchasing and storeroom personnel help assure that the correct supplies are available. They also assure supplies have been stored and handled correctly to maintain their potency and purity, and should assist in the removal of expired supplies.

The most important support for compounding personnel is other IV admixtures personnel. The IV room supervising pharmacist helps prevent medication errors by cross-checking additive labels, orders, plunger positions, compounder settings, calculations and documentation. The supervisor and other compounding personnel also observe your gowning, materials set-up, selection of tools, and your manipulative technique. Heavy workloads may encourage haste and short-cuts on the part of the even the most dedicated personnel. We may all need a gentle reminder from time to time. All personnel on the IV team must cultivate the ability both **to point out errors** without causing offense, and to **accept constructive criticism** without taking offense; a kind of IV "honor system".

Many pressures and distractions can lead to errors which may cause harm or death. By sharing responsibility, all personnel involved in compounding can gain additional assurance they have not inadvertently harmed a patient.

Self-evaluation: Quality Assurance Theory for IV Admixtures

1. The most common cause of contamination is _____.
   (Page 3)

2. Quality Assurance (QA) relies primarily upon product testing to assure product quality. (Pages 4, 5, and 6)

                                 True   False

3. Substances which cause disease are called _____.
   (Pages 2 and 3)

4. Substances which cause inflammation are called _____.
   (Pages 2 and 4)

5. Cross-contamination can occur when _____.
   (Pages 1 and 4)

6. In a QA approach to monitoring, end-product testing demonstrates that the process is operating within _____.
   (Page 6)

7. The system of controls and practices used to prevent contamination when compounding drugs is called _____. (Pages 1 and 2)

8. The body's natural routes of absorption are through the _____, _____, and _____. (Page 2)

9. Administration of medications by hypodermic injection is a form of _____ route administration, which quickly spreads pain-relieving and disease-fighting drugs throughout the body. (Page i and 2)

10. Engineering controls limit contamination _____. (Page 6)

11. Barrier controls limit contamination_____ .(Page 6)

12. Aseptic manipulative techniques limit contamination_____.
    (Page 7)

13. The key component in assuring the quality of IV admixtures is the _____, supported by a _____.
    (Pages 7 and 8)

II. ENGINEERING CONTROLS AND LAMINAR AIRFLOW THEORY

LEARNING OBJECTIVES FOR SECTION II.

Upon completion of this section, you should be able to perform the following tasks:

Objective 2.1) Understand and define Primary and Secondary Engineering Controls.

Objective 2.2) Understand and define the use of the HEPA filter.

Objective 2.3) Understand and define the use of laminar airflow.

Objective 2.4) Diagram the airflow patterns in a Laminar Flow Cleanbench (LFCB).

Objective 2.5) Describe the limitations of the LFCB, and its contamination models.

Objective 2.6) Diagram the airflow patterns in a Biological Safety Cabinet (BSC), and determine where air can be expected to be: a) clean, b) microbiologically contaminated, and c) contaminated with residual drug product.

Objective 2.7) Describe the limitations of the BSC, and list practices which defeat its protective qualities.

Objective 2.8) Describe the design characteristics of the Buffer Zone, and its function in IV compounding procedures.

Objective 2.9) Describe the function of anterooms or gowning areas.

TERMS FOR SECTION II

Biological Safety Cabinet (BioSafety Cabinet, BSC)	A specially-designed workbench providing both product and operator protection in which HEPA-filtered "laminar" air flows vertically from above the work zone, toward the work surface ***and is recovered.***

Critical Site	Any direct pathway through which contaminants may enter a sterile product.
First Air	Unobstructed air issuing directly from the HEPA filter.
HEPA Filter	**H**igh **E**fficiency **P**articulate **A**ir Filter capable of removing at least 99.97% of particles larger or smaller than 0.3 microns from the air.
Hood	A term used for specially-designed enclosures wherein airflow is controlled to provide a variety of conditions for critical processes. Included are Horizontal Flow Cleanbenches (HFCBs), Biological Safety Cabinets (BSCs), Vertical Flow Cleanbenches (VFCBs) and Chemical Fume Hoods (CFHs). (CFHs provide user protection, only, and are rarely used in pharmacy.)
Horizontal Flow Cleanbench (HFCB)	A specially-designed workbench in which HEPA-filtered "laminar" air flows horizontally from the rear to the front opening of the hood, where it exits to the environment. It provides product protection, only.
Laminar Airflow	This term has been traditionally used to describe the airflow in Cleanbenches and certain Cleanrooms, but is technically incorrect. The correct terms are either "unidirectional airflow", or "columnated airflow". We will, however, follow convention and use the term Laminar Airflow, which is defined as air flowing in one direction, at a uniform speed.
Laminar Flow Cleanbench (LFCB)	A general term that includes the HFCB, and VFCB, where air exits directly to the environment.
Smoke-split	The region where air descending from the HEPA filter of a BSC splits, with part of the air exiting through the front grill, and part through the rear grill or slots.
Vertical Flow Cleanbench (VFCB)	Although some of the air in a BSC flows vertically, not all vertical flow hoods are BSCs. Vertical Flow Cleanbenches simply supply HEPA-filtered air from the top of the hood (rather than the rear of the hood, as in an HFCB). They

do not recover contaminated air as is the case in a BSC. Remember: the VFCB provides **product protection,** only.

Objective 2.1) Understand and define Primary and Secondary Engineering Controls.

Key Concept: Engineering controls reduce **contamination potential** by limiting the amount of contaminants in, and near the work environment. **Primary engineering controls** (hoods) are used to create the work zone in which aseptic processing is conducted. **Secondary engineering controls** provide a buffer zone (sometimes called the core) in which the hoods are located, and an anteroom, or gowning area between the buffer zone and the uncontrolled general environment.

The purpose of the buffer zone (or core) is to limit general atmospheric and surface contamination levels, thus reducing the risk of contamination of the aseptic work zone. The anteroom, or gowning area, provides a clean zone in which gowning is donned and removed, and working materials are removed from outer wrappings and pre-cleaned before transfer to the buffer zone.

Objective 2.2) Understand and define the use of the HEPA filter.

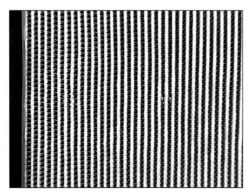

Figure 1. The HEPA filter.

Key Concept: High Efficiency Particulate Air (HEPA) filters remove virtually all particles from the air.

HEPA filters remove 99.97% (or more, depending upon the rating of the HEPA filter) of particulates larger (and smaller) than 0.3 μm (micrometer, micron). Different forces result in the removal of larger particles and smaller particles. On the average, 0.3 μm particles are the least-efficiently removed by either set of forces. For this reason, filters are rated and tested at this "worst case" particle size[5].

HEPA-filtered air is virtually free of **airborne** microbial and other particulate contaminants. Provided that contaminants are not introduced on work materials or by the operator, the use of HEPA-filtered air in Laminar Flow Cleanbenches (LFCBs) produces a work environment that is free from airborne contaminants. This is **all** it does. HEPA-filtered air may pick up contaminants from dirty items in its path, but **it will not disinfect or sterilize those items.**

The HEPA filter is delicate, and easily damaged. Nothing should be allowed to touch the filter, or be squirted or splattered into it. The pleats on most HEPA filters are separated by strips of aluminum.. The filter may, or may not have a protective screen in front of it. In either case, if pressure is applied to the aluminum separators or the screen, the separators may cause leakage by penetrating the back side of the filter medium pleat. Such damage is often irreparable and can only be detected by testing.

FIRST AIR

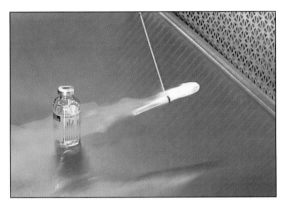

First air is clean air issuing directly from the HEPA filter, with no obstruction in its path. All critical sites and critical manipulations must be carried out in the flow of "first air". The operator must apply the "first air" concept to all critical sites and pathways.

Figure 2. First air flow in a Horizontal Flow Cleanbench

Objective 2.3) Understand and define the use of laminar (unidirectional) airflow.

Key Concept: Laminar airflow is air flowing in a single direction at a uniform speed. These characteristics produce a cohesive wash of clean air, without eddies or cross-currents. When HEPA-filtered air is supplied in this manner, contaminated air is pushed out of the work zone, and room air is prevented from freely entering the front opening of the hood.

Because the flow of air in an LFCB is relatively slow **(90 feet per minute ± 20%)**, this wash of clean air is easily disrupted. Air currents caused by ventilation or activities in the room, rapid and erratic motions by the operator, objects blocking the uniform flow of air, speaking, laughing, etc., can all disrupt the laminar flow of HEPA-filtered air, leading to contamination (and, in the case of the BSC used to compound hazardous substances, can cause operator and environmental exposure to hazardous drugs).

Objective 2.4) Describe the airflow patterns of the Laminar Flow Cleanbench (LFCB).

Key Concept: Clean, HEPA-filtered "first air", which is virtually free of particulate contaminants, is supplied to the work zone to reduce the risk of product contamination from **airborne sources** _only._ The clean "first air" is supplied horizontally from a supply HEPA filter at the back of the Horizontal LFCB, and flows from back to front. First air flows from a supply HEPA filter above the work zone in a Vertical LFCB, and turns horizontally at the worksurface to flow out through the front of the unit.

**Remember: a VFCB and a Biological Safety Cabinet (BSC) are not the same. A VFCB is not suitable for compounding hazardous substances.**

Objective 2.5) Describe the limitations of the LFCB, and its contamination models.

Key Concept: The LFCB provides only a work environment that is easy to clean and is supplied with a relatively slow-moving wash of clean air. The LFCB must be properly cleaned and disinfected, and the following types of contamination prevented:

> **Backwash Contamination**
> **Downstream Contamination**
> **Cross-stream Contamination**

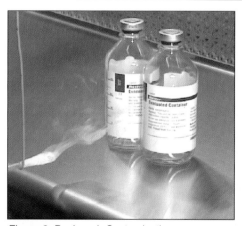

Figure 3. Backwash Contamination

Backwash contamination may occur if room air washes back into the front opening of the LFCB. It should be assumed, under normal operating conditions, that air in the front six inches of the LFCB is intermittently contaminated in this way. Also, excessive or erratic movements, traffic, and ventilation systems immediately in front of the LFCB may result in the influx of room air to the critical work zone. Items placed into the hood may also create a **zone of confusion** extending toward the front of the hood as much as **six** times the diameter of the object, if it has laminar flow on one side (i.e. objects immediately adjacent to the hood wall), and **three** times the object diameter if it is exposed to laminar flow **on both sides.** This also can contribute to backwash contamination.

Downstream contamination occurs when the air passes over non-sterile objects, picking up contamination which may then be carried to critical sites downstream from the objects. All critical sites must be kept in "first air" throughout the compounding process. Items should be arranged single-file, parallel to the filter in an HFCB (Horizontal Flow Cleanbench).

Cross-stream contamination occurs when disturbances or eddies are created in the hood, causing air to carry contaminants from one item to another. Rapid hand movements, overcrowding of supplies, and improper placement of critical sites relative to equipment may result in such eddies in the airflow.

Objective 2.6) Describe the airflow patterns of the BSC.

NOTE: *This manual is not designed to provide a complete discussion of hazardous substance compounding. The design and use of the BSC, and some general rules for handling hazardous substances are included here because many pharmacies use Biological Safety Cabinets for compounding substances other than chemotherapeutic agents. It is recommended that all personnel engaged in chemotherapeutic agent compounding undergo thorough training in their institution's procedures for safe handling of chemotherapeutic agents, and be validated in their technique for this application.*

Key Concept: The BSC is designed to provide a wash of clean air to the critical work surface for product protection. It also recovers potentially contaminated air from the work space for personnel protection, and then HEPA-filters this recovered air to prevent the introduction of hazardous particulates to the environment. When properly used, the BSC provides product protection from airborne particulate contaminants, and protection of personnel and the environment from hazardous particulates.

There are several types of BSC, with different configurations for specific uses. **It is important that the type of hood used is matched to the specific application.** Almost all pharmacy BSCs are Class II. Class II is further subdivided into types.

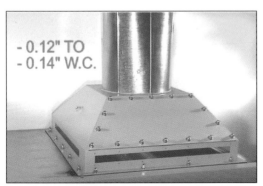

- 0.12" TO
- 0.14" W.C.

Figure 4. A negative pressure exhaust duct is required for materials which produce hazardous fumes or vapors.

Type A and Type B3 are similar in that approximately 30% of the internal air is vented through an exhaust HEPA filter, and 70% is recirculated through the supply HEPA filter. The difference is that the B3 is connected to the outside via negatively pressurized ducts, facilitating complete removal of **small amounts** of hazardous vapors and fumes from the work zone. The Type A is exhausted into the room, and does not contain or remove any hazardous fumes or gases. The Type B3 cannot be used for large amounts of hazardous fumes because

70% of the air is recirculated, which may allow fume build-up to occur[6]. Most pharmacy hoods are Class II, Type A/B3 convertible designs.

The Class II, Type B2 BSC is known as a **"total exhaust"** hood, because 100% of internal air is exhausted through negative pressure ducts to the outside, preventing the build-up of hazardous fumes. Note that Type B2 and B3 hoods must be vented via **negative pressure ducts.** If positive pressure develops in the ducts, fumes or gases can be forced out into the environment and back pressure on the exhaust filter may interfere with proper hood operation[6].

AIRFLOW PATTERNS IN THE BIOLOGICAL SAFETY CABINET

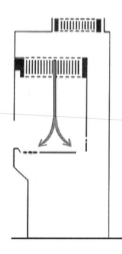

1. HEPA-Filtered Supply Air

In a BSC, HEPA-filtered "first air", which is virtually free of particulate contaminants, is supplied to the work zone. This provides an environment in which aseptic compounding procedures may be performed, thus reducing the risk of product contamination from airborne sources. The clean "first air" is supplied vertically downward from a supply HEPA filter located above the work zone.

Figure 5. Down-flowing Supply Air.

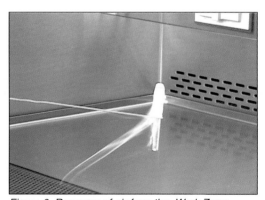

Figure 6. Recovery of air from the Work Zone

2. Recovery of Work Zone Air

As the air approaches the work surface it "splits" and turns in its directional flow, with a portion of the air exiting through a grill at the front of the cabinet, and the rest exiting through a grill at the rear of the work surface (in some BSCs the back grill is a series of holes in the back wall of the cabinet). Air which has passed through the work zone may be contaminated with hazardous drugs.

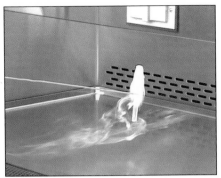

The area where the air separates, known as the **"smoke-split"**, can be visualized with smoke. A **"Zone of Confusion"** exists in the center of the smoke-split (along a lateral line approximately mid-worksurface). Work should not be carried out directly under the smoke-split. It is best to work behind the smoke-split, since contaminated air from this area is carried through the back grill of the cabinet.

Figure 7. "Smoke-split" showing the "Zone of Confusion"

3. Recirculation and Exhaust of Recovered Air

Internal air drawn from the smoke-split to the front and back of the cabinet traverses the undertray area, and returns to the top of the cabinet, where a portion is recirculated through the supply HEPA filter, and a portion is exhausted through an exhaust HEPA filter. This exhausted air is replaced by incoming air at the face of the BSC. (There is no recirculation in a Type B2, but the general operational principles are the same.) The exhaust HEPA filter helps protect the environment from contamination with hazardous particulate substances. Negative pressure ducting may be incorporated to recover fumes and vapors.

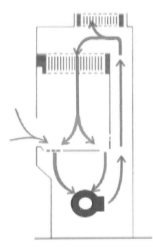

Figure 8. BSC internal airflow patterns

4. Make-up Air Provides Containment

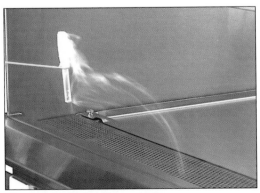

Figure 9. In-flowing Make-up Air

"Make-up" room air, which replaces the exhausted volume, is drawn into the front of the cabinet and down through the front grill, providing an in-flowing barrier of air. This in-flowing air helps contain hazardous substances liberated in the work zone, providing protection for the environment and the operator.

CONTAMINATION WITHIN THE BIOLOGICAL SAFETY CABINET

Air may become contaminated with hazardous drug as it passes through the work zone, and may contain droplets or particles of drug that have escaped from the vial or ampule during manipulations. This air should be considered to be contaminated with hazardous drugs. Because some of this contaminated air passes forward through the front grill and through the undertray area, **these areas must also be considered to be contaminated with hazardous drugs.** Air passing through the work zone may also become contaminated with pyrogenic, pathogenic, and other particulate matter introduced on the operator's gloves and sleeves, or on compounding materials. **Remember: *aseptic manipulations must always be carried out in first air.***

Room air drawn through the front opening is contaminated with viable and non-viable particulates. Air near the opening of the hood, as far back from the grill as three inches, may contain particulates carried in from the room. This air is also drawn through the front grill and undertray area, which must be considered to be contaminated. **The undertray area requires regular, frequent cleaning and disinfection.**

Objective 2.7) Describe the limitations of the BSC and list practices which defeat its protective qualities.

Key Concept: Airflow in a BSC is relatively slow and may be defeated. The protective characteristics of a BSC derive from the fact that the air is moving in a uniform direction at a uniform speed (Laminar Airflow). Anything that disrupts this flow can create eddies that may carry contaminants to the product or hazardous drugs out into the environment. Because the airflow is relatively slow, it may easily be disrupted in any of the following ways:

1. Items placed in the path of the first air will disturb the laminar flow, as will rapid or erratic hand movements.

2. Sources of air movement outside the cabinet, such as traffic, air-conditioning, or ventilation systems may also effect the airflow pattern in the front portion of the BSC, as may the operator's arms extending into the BSC.

3. Items placed on the front return grill will prevent in-flowing room air and out-flowing work zone air from being properly recovered. Items placed on or against the rear return grills will also inhibit recovery of air from the work zone.

4. Air currents produced by talking, laughing or sneezing move much more rapidly than first air from a HEPA filter, and can readily defeat it. Also, air that is

under pressure, such as air escaping from a vial, or spray produced when an ampule is opened or a needle is crushed or broken may overcome the protective airflow in a BSC, momentarily allowing the escape of contaminants.

5. Improper adjustment of the sash height will change the velocity of in-flowing air, relative to down-flowing air, as well as the laminar downflow profile quality. If the inflow velocity is too low, **contaminated air may escape into the environment.** If it is too high, **dirty room air may flow into the work zone**, compromising product sterility. Always set the front sash to the marked height (usually 8").

6. The BSC should operate twenty-four hours a day, seven days a week. It has been suggested by some sources that turning the BSC off without proper preparation and sealing may allow contaminated air from the undertray and plenum areas of the cabinet to escape into the room. If it is absolutely necessary to turn the unit off for any period, professional Safety advice should be obtained[7].

7. The BSC should be performance-tested by qualified personnel at least annually, preferably every 6 months. Because the air circulation patterns of the BSC are complex, and the protective characteristics of the cabinet are dependent on both the integrity of the HEPA filters and the maintenance of proper velocities, the unit should be routinely tested for proper performance upon installation, every 6 months[8], and whenever it is moved. **Velocities change as the filters load with contaminants.**

A BSC may require testing when repairs are made that require opening non-user accessible portions of the cabinet, following repairs or adjustments required due to ingress of debris, or when other signs of malfunction are observed. **No attempt to adjust the velocities or repair a BSC should ever be made by the user.**

Objective 2.8) Describe the design characteristics of the Buffer Zone, and its function in IV compounding procedures.

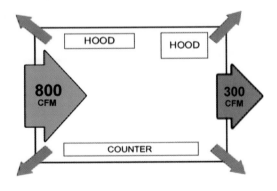

Key Concept: Because the design limitations of hoods may allow room air to enter the work zone, and contaminants may be introduced when materials are placed in the hood, it is desirable to provide a buffer zone around the hood where contaminants are limited to the greatest extent possible.

Figure 10 . Pressurization causes air to flow outward, from cleaner areas to dirtier areas.

Ideally, the buffer zone is supplied with HEPA-filtered air, usually in a conventional flow (non-laminar) arrangement. A sufficient quantity of air is supplied to produce a specified level of air cleanliness. **For pharmacy operations this is usually Class 10,000 or Class 100,000. This means that there are no more than 10,000 or 100,000 particles 0.5 μm or larger per cubic foot of air, respectively** [9,10]. In some states, a class 1,000 cleanroom may be required.

It is also desirable to keep the buffer zone at a higher pressure than the anteroom, which is, in turn, at a higher pressure than the general environment. This arrangement prevents particles from infiltrating through seams, and causes air to flow outward, from cleaner to dirtier areas when doors are opened. Positive pressurization of a closed space is created by supplying more air than is removed from the room through return ducts and exfiltration.

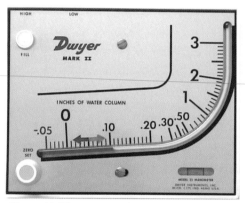

Figure 11. Water manometers can be used to verify correct operating pressures.

Pressurized facilities are often equipped with magnihelic gauges or inclined water manometers to verify proper pressurization. If your facility is designed in this way, learn the pressure specifications and document the readings on a pressurization log each time you use the rooms. Loss of pressure may indicate a problem with the air supply system, or loading of HEPA filters [5,6].

Some cleanroom complexes are equipped with **pass-through boxes** for introducing supplies and removing product and waste materials. When passing through the anteroom, or using pass-through boxes, only one door should be opened at a time. This procedure is designed to maintain room pressure, keeping contaminants out of the buffer zone surrounding the critical work zones within the hoods.

Buffer zones, anterooms, and other controlled facilities are also designed to be easily cleaned. The environmental surfaces should be hard, smooth, and resistant to damage from cleaning and disinfectant compounds. Ledges, seams, and crevices should be minimized, and wire shelving used to prevent surface dust accumulation[5,9].

Housekeeping procedures should be **in writing,** and their performance should be **documented** on a housekeeping or sanitizing log to assure the cleanest possible environment[5,9].

Objective 2.9) Describe the function of anterooms or gowning areas.

Key Concept: Anterooms or gowning areas are transition areas for **gowning, de-gowning and materials staging and preparation.**

If the IV room or buffer zone door opens into the general environment, gowning will be donned in an uncontrolled area, and may become contaminated before entry into the buffer zone. Contaminants may also be transferred directly from the core to the outside environment. Likewise, materials removed from outer shipping containers and wrappers prior to transfer to the buffer zone will be unprotected from uncontrolled levels of airborne and surface contaminants. A separate gowning area or anteroom provides a place for these activities that has a controlled level of potential contaminants, and thus helps progressively minimize the amount of contamination introduced into the buffer zone, or core[4,5,9].

Self-evaluation: Engineering Controls

1. Clean air issuing directly from the HEPA filter is called _____. (Pages 11 and 13)

2. Laminar-flowing air moves at a uniform _____ in a uniform _____. (Pages 11 and 13)

3. A laminar flow clean bench helps reduce the risk of contamination from _____ sources. (Pages 12 and 14)

4. _____ contamination may occur within the front 6 inches of an LFCB when disruptive activities occur outside the hood. (Page 14)

5. _____ contamination occurs when contaminants are picked up from objects in the path of the first air and carried to an object further from the HEPA filter. (Page 14)

6. _____ contamination occurs when contaminants are carried from side to side in the hood because of eddies created in the airflow by disruptive motions or crowded items. (Page 15)

7. In a BSC, air flowing vertically from above the work zone splits as it approaches the work surface, with part of the air exiting through the front grills and part through the back. This area is called the _____. (Pages 11 and 17)

8. _____ (Choose One) Work should be not carried out:

a) in front of,

b) directly under, or

c) behind the area described in number 7. (Page 17)

9. When working in a BSC, the front sash should be lowered as far as possible. (Page 19)   True   False

10. Air in a Laminar Flow cleanbench moves at about _____ feet per minute. (Page 13)

11. The two types of engineering controls used to support the aseptic process are:_____ and_____ engineering controls. (Page 12)

12. The Vertical Flow Clean Bench is used for compounding hazardous materials. (Pages 11, 12 and 14)   True   False

13. Putting pressure on the HEPA filter may drive the _____ _____ through the filtration medium at the rear of the filter. (Page 13)

14. The LFCB is a _____ Engineering Control. (Page 12)

15. The HEPA filter retains _____% of contaminants larger and smaller than 0.3μm in diameter. (Pages 11, 12 and 14)

16. In a Biological Safety Cabinet, a _____ of _____ exists in the smoke-split area. (Page 17)

17. In a horizontal LFCB, all working materials should be arranged front to back. (Page 14)   True   False

18. Pressurization of a cleanroom causes air to flow from _____ to_____ areas. (Pages 19 and 20)

19. A properly operating BSC will contain all hazardous contaminants and completely prevent contamination of the environment and personnel. (Pages 18 and 19)   True   False

20. Air flowing from the front of a HFCB has sufficient velocity to prevent the entry of contaminants into the work zone under almost all circumstances. (Page 14)   True   False

III. BARRIER CONTROLS

LEARNING OBJECTIVES FOR SECTION III.

Upon completion of this section you should be able to:

Objective 3.1) Describe the function of various barrier controls in aseptic processing and hazardous materials compounding.

Objective 3.2) Properly use, remove, and dispose of barrier controls for aseptic processing and hazardous materials compounding.

TERMS FOR SECTION III.

Bacteriostatic   Preventing the growth or multiplication of bacteria.

Bioburden   The level of microorganisms present as potential contaminants. (The higher the level of bioburden, the more difficult it is to achieve or maintain sterility.)

Chemotherapeutic Agent   This term means chemicals systematically administered for the treatment of microbial infection, although it is often improperly associated with the treatment of cancer. Another common term employed is *cytotoxic agent (CYTA)* which means *toxic to cells*. A third term is *oncolytic,* which means *tumor-dissolving*. A fourth term is *antineoplastic,* which means *against new growth*. Technically, none of these terms is exclusively linked to cancer treatment (not all tumors and neoplasms are malignant), and many other diseases are treated with the types of drugs usually associated with these terms. The term *hazardous substance* or hazardous materials, with certain limitations (see next definition) is preferred, but this manual occasionally defaults to common usage for clarity (for example chemo-gowns are not called hazardous-substances gowns)

Hazardous Substances (Materials, Drugs)   A term applied to particularly hazardous drugs. All drugs are employed because they have physiological effects, therefore none can be considered to be completely safe, in any amount, under all circumstances. Care should be taken to minimize unnecessary exposure to any drug product. However, certain drugs are known to be **carcinogens, teratogens, mutagens, are toxic in very small amounts, or produce toxic vapors.** Such drugs require special precautions and are hazardous under all circumstances of exposure. They are not always anti-cancer drugs. Many antivirals, immune suppressants and other drugs fall into this category.

Sloughing   Shedding of dead skin cells and debris from the surface of the skin.

Objective 3.1) Describe the function of various barrier controls in aseptic processing and hazardous materials compounding.

Key Concept: Gowning serves as a barrier which reduces the risk of transferring contaminants from skin, hair, and clothing to the product. In the case of hazardous substances, it also reduces the risk of personnel exposure, and of the transfer of contaminants to the general environment.

The following barrier controls are recommended, and support protection of the product, personnel, and the environment, as noted. If you do not use all items described, you should understand the increased risks, and adjust your work practices accordingly.

HAIR COVER: A hair cover is worn to prevent sloughing of contamination such as hair, dandruff, and bacteria from the head into the work area. This also applies to personnel who are bald, because the skin of the scalp sheds, whether hair is present, or not. When compounding hazardous substances, the head cover also reduces the likelihood that contaminants will be carried to the hair. Pushing uncovered hair back from the face is a common, unconscious gesture, which can transfer contaminants to or from the hair. As with all barrier controls, head covers are to be worn intact, as designed. **(Provides product and personnel protection)**

FACE MASK: A face mask is worn to contain droplets of saliva generated during speech, coughing, laughing, or other activities, and to reduce their introduction to the work area. It is recommended that all personnel wear face masks at all times while compounding. Personnel with active allergies should be especially careful to use masks, however, personnel with upper respiratory infections or colds should not compound. If face masks do not cover all facial hair, a beard cover should be worn. Face masks should cover the nose, be properly fastened, and be fitted over the bridge of the nose. **(Provides product protection)**

GOWN: A gown is worn to prevent shedding of particles from the operator's clothing and exposed skin onto the work area. The gown also serves as a barrier, protecting personnel from hazardous drug particles. When compounding hazardous substances, it is recommended that the gown be back-closing, with long, cuffed sleeves, and be made of low-absorbency material. **(Provides product, personnel, and environmental protection)**

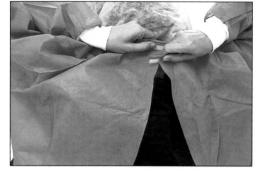

Figure 12. Gowns worn for compounding hazardous substances should be back-closing, with long, cuffed sleeves.

GLOVES: Gloves are worn both to reduce the possibility of touch contamination, and to protect the individual from coming into contact with harmful compounds. **(Provide product and personnel protection).**

GOGGLES: Protective goggles are worn when compounding hazardous substances to prevent splashing or squirting harmful substances into the eyes. **(Provide personnel protection)**

SHOE COVERS: Shoe covers are worn in the IV room to contain contamination carried in (or out, in the case of hazardous materials) on the shoes, especially the soles. **(Provide product, personnel and environmental protection)**

Objective 3.2) Properly use, remove, and dispose of barrier controls for aseptic processing and hazardous materials compounding.

Key Concept: Barrier controls can reduce the transfer of contaminants both to, and from the compounding area. However, if improperly used, the purpose of barrier items may be defeated, and they may actually contribute to contamination of product or transfer of contaminants to the operator or environment.

Gowning should be donned from the top down, with gloves donned last. Do not allow gowning to drag on the floor. If your anteroom is equipped with a gowning bench, don all gowning except gloves and shoe covers. Sit on the bench with feet on the dirty (outer) side and put on shoe covers, moving each shoe, as it is covered, to the clean side of the bench. Don and prepare gloves.

All barriers should be worn intact, as they were designed to be worn. All ties and fasteners are to be fastened properly, and where possible, adjusted to the operator. The following specific procedures should be observed:

HYGIENE: Prior to gloving, wash hands and forearms thoroughly using hand soap which does not interfere with skin pH. Particular attention should be given to the fingernails. This procedure helps reduce bioburden on the skin and thus reduces the possibility of **touch** contamination. The use of harsh cleaning agents is <u>not</u> recommended because they have not been demonstrated to enhance the effectiveness of the glove barrier, and because such agents may cause skin irritation or contribute to the development of sensitivity.

Washing removes only the **transient flora** on the surface of the skin, which represent about **15%** of the flora present. Regardless of the type of cleanser used, or the intensity of scrubbing, human skin will always harbor **resident flora** such as bacteria and other microorganisms in the pores and follicles, which constitute **85%** of the bioburden on skin and begin replenishing transient flora immediately[11].

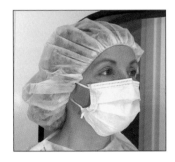

USE OF FACE MASKS: Fit face masks properly to your face, covering the nose, and tie both the top and bottom ties, if using tie-back masks. Dispose of face masks upon removal. Do not allow them to lie about, because they are concentrated sources of potentially infectious agents, and are highly unsavory to your co-workers.

USE OF GOWNS: Gowns should not be worn outside the anteroom or compounding area. Wearing gowns in general areas defeats the purpose of their use, which is to limit the transfer of environmental contaminants to the work area. In the case of chemo-gowns, the gown is also designed to prevent the transfer of hazardous materials to both the operator and the environment. It must be assumed that at least the lower portion of the chemo-gown sleeve is contaminated during the compounding process. Therefore, the chemo-gown should be removed in a manner that contains any contaminants and disposed of immediately upon completion of compounding.

To do this, remove outer gloves properly (see below) and unfasten the gown closures. Grasp the back shoulder area of the gown with the opposite hand and pull the gown forward over the sleeve. Secure the covered sleeve through the gown fabric and remove the arm. Repeat this procedure for the other side, to contain any contaminants on the sleeves or outer surfaces of the gown, which should now be inside-out. Chemo gowns should not be reused or worn outside the compounding area.

Do not store or reuse gowns used for compounding hazardous substances.

USE OF GLOVES: Gloves should fit properly. Personnel who are sensitive to latex now have many non-latex and non-powdered options, available in a full range of sizes.

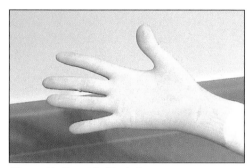
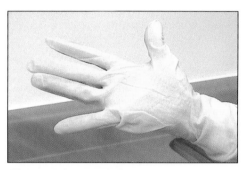

Figure 13. Properly fitted gloves.   *Figure 14. Improperly fitted gloves.*

Loose gloves tear easily and may interfere with manipulative technique, thus compromising either product quality, user safety, or both.

Gloves should never be considered to be sterile. Because the operator handles numerous non-sterile items during the compounding process, contamination of the glove surface is inevitable. Gloves do, however, help to contain sloughing from the skin, and should be periodically disinfected with 70% alcohol to reduce bioburden and achieve hand-surface bacteriostasis. **Gloves are <u>not</u> a substitute for proper manipulative technique.** Conversely, proper manipulative technique cannot prevent natural sloughing from the exposed skin of ungloved hands.

New <u>**latex**</u> gloves have been shown to **transfer 175 particles** ≥5µm per square centimeter of surface touched, while the **rate of transfer was reduced to 3 particles after washing.** A similar study of <u>**nitrile**</u> gloves showed that new gloves **transferred 1000 to 4000 particles** of ≥0.5µm per square centimeter of surface touched, while **the level after washing was 25 to 100 particles.** Washing gloves after donning also removes lubricant powders added during their manufacture[12].

The powder and particles on gloves can easily be transferred to septa, and then into solutions as the needle passes into the vial. Even if the gloves are initially sterile, they do not remain so, and the powder may be pyrogenic, and often contains latex from the glove surface, which may be a potent allergen. After washing, **gloves are to be disinfected with 70% alcohol, and allowed to dry in the laminar airflow slipstream, prior to compounding.** This procedure assures a bacteriostatic surface for the hands and eliminates the effects of sloughing. Gloves should also be **re-rinsed with 70% alcohol each time the individual enters the critical work zone and frequently, throughout compounding.**

Gloves can be penetrated by certain substances over time, and may become torn. It has been found that many gloves tested after 2 hours of use had unnoticed pin-holes[12]. When compounding hazardous materials, double-gloving and frequent changing of gloves is recommended. Double gloving provides additional protection from penetration or tears, and permits the operator to remove contaminated, possibly dripping, outer gloves immediately in the event of a spill without leaving the hands unprotected. In this procedure the gloves should be donned so that the first pair lies inside and under the sleeve cuff. The second pair should then be placed over the cuff. This provides a better barrier against contaminant transfer to the skin.

The outer gloves are to be removed and discarded whenever the operator's hands are removed from the hood, to avoid carrying contaminants to furniture, storage bins, supplies, doorknobs, telephones, computer keyboards, pens, and numerous other items outside the hood. Recent studies have demonstrated contamination of the general environment with chemotherapeutic agents, and have also detected mutagenic effects in personnel responsible for compounding and administering hazardous substances, **even when the Biological Safety Cabinets used in compounding were found to be operating properly and the operator was wearing gloves.** Most of this contamination is attributable to poor technique, inadequate cleaning of hoods, and transfer of contaminants on product, gloves and other gowning items to the environment[13].

DE-GLOVING PROCEDURE

De-glove the outer pair by grasping one glove on the outside and pulling the glove off, inside out, reducing it to a ball in the opposite hand. Slip the fingers of the hand from which the outer glove was removed under the cuff of the remaining outer glove. Pull the remaining outer glove down and over the balled glove, taking care not to contaminate either inner glove, turning the glove inside out as it encloses the first glove.

Grasp the inside surface of the second glove, which is now the outer surface of the ball, securing the outer gloves inside-out, with all contamination inside the ball, and dispose of in the BSC internal waste container. Remove the hands from the BSC, don and wash a fresh pair of outer gloves, and disinfect with 70% isopropyl alcohol before returning to compounding. If compounding is completed, remove the gown next, followed by remaining items of gowning. Then remove the inner pair of gloves in the same manner as the outer pair. Dispose of all materials in a Chemo Waste container.

Self-evaluation: Barrier Controls

1. If the operator has not spilled anything while compounding hazardous substances, gowns may be carefully stored in the compounding area, and reused for one shift, only. (Pages 26 and 27)

    True   False

2. Gloves are sterile barriers to contamination of the IV admixture. (Page 27)

    True   False

3. It is acceptable to wear barrier controls outside the compounding area, provided these barriers are not used in compounding hazardous substances. (Page 26)

    True   False

4. Each time the operator leaves the aseptic field, gloves need to be disinfected before reentering the aseptic field. (Page 28)

    True   False

5. Name four barrier controls _____, _____, _____, and _____. (Pages 24 and 25)

6. Barriers used in compounding hazardous substances should be used only once, and must be de-gowned in accordance with special procedures. (Pages 26, 27 and 28)

    True   False

7. New, unpowdered gloves are virtually particulate-free. (Page 27)

    True   False

8. It is acceptable to tear a small hole in the back of the hair cover for heat relief. (Page 26)

    True   False

IV. ASEPTIC MANIPULATIONS

LEARNING OBJECTIVES FOR SECTION IV.

Upon completion of this section you should be able to explain the reasons for the following procedures and perform them consistently:

Objective 4.1) Prepare equipment and facilities, and pre-stage working materials.

Objective 4.2) Prepare hoods for aseptic compounding.

Objective 4.3) Stage materials for compounding in the hood correctly.

Objective 4.4) Properly arrange material in the work space.

Objective 4.5) Select the appropriate compounding tools for each task.

Objective 4.6) Evaluate risk factors, correctly perform core manipulative techniques used for various component packaging systems and devices, and understand the methods to be used in developing compounding procedures.

TERMS FOR SECTION IV.

Alcohol	Alcohol is a **non-polar** solvent which is used as a disinfectant. Acceptable alcohols are Isopropyl alcohol (IPA) and Ethanol (EtOH). In both cases, the most effective concentration of alcohol in deionized (DI) water is 70%.
Bevel	The angled portion of the needle tip, which produces a sharp point.
Core	A small particle of rubber broken away and carried into the drug solution as the needle penetrates the rubber closure.
Hydrophilic	"Water-loving". This term applies to the air filtration medium of many dispensing pins, which allows both liquids and air to pass through.

Hydrophobic	"Water-fearing". This term applies to the air filtration medium of dispensing pins designed for hazardous substances, which allows air to pass, but not liquids.
Luer-Lok™	A proprietary system incorporating a spiral locking collar into which the needle hub is inserted, and turned to lock the needle securely in place.
Lumen	The hole running through the center of the needle cannula.
Plasmolysis	Dissolution of the microbial cell wall, causing the disintegration of the cell and death of the organism.

Because it is not possible to present procedures for every compounding task or item of equipment you may encounter, you should understand the methods used to develop procedures, and the system employed by pharmacy to validate them. Validation of pharmacy operations occurs on two levels: 1) Technique Validation, and 2) Process Validation. **Technique Validation** demonstrates the ability of the operator to perform fundamental core manipulative techniques. **Process Validation** demonstrates the suitability of the application of these core techniques to a specific compounding process. When developing new techniques or processes, you should apply your knowledge of contamination sources, engineering controls, and barrier controls to the physical manipulation of drug products. **An evaluation of the risks** presented by each operation and **development of a plan for achieving quality** in each product are integral to good aseptic technique. All pharmacy procedures should be in writing.

Objective 4.1) Prepare equipment and facilities, and pre-stage working materials.

Key Concept: Because the compounding environment must meet validation conditions for the process to be performed consistently in accordance with established procedures, the operator must assure that all equipment is functioning properly, all barrier controls are in place, and all materials required for the process are in place and meet criteria.

KEEPING THE COMPOUNDING ENVIRONMENT CLEAN

Under no circumstances should food or drink be brought into any compounding area, or stored in an area or refrigerator dedicated to the storage of drugs.

Cardboard (corrugate) boxes, paper wrappers, and street clothes are all excellent sources of particulate contamination. To minimize particulate introduction into the buffer zone, personnel should cover their street clothes, (or scrubs, if they are worn outside the compounding area), with low-linting barrier controls. All packaging materials not required to maintain sterility should be removed in the anteroom. Any dust or overt soiling should be wiped from bottles, vials, ampules, bags and other supplies with a low-lint wipe, moistened with 70% IPA. Use care to avoid damaging labels.

All jewelry must be removed from hands and wrists because it cannot be adequately cleaned or disinfected, and can also become contaminated with hazardous substances. It is recommended that no rings, earrings, necklaces, watches, or bracelets be worn. Makeup and nail polish are also sources of contamination and should not be worn when compounding.

Sometimes, a **"tacky mat"** is placed at the entrance to the buffer zone. A tacky mat consists of several layers of sticky plastic sheets, which will pull dust and dirt from the wheels of carts and the bottoms of shoes. If you have a tacky mat, be sure you step on it with both feet, and roll all cart wheels across it. The tacky mat should be renewed at the beginning of each shift. To renew the clean surface, simply peel away the top layer of the mat and dispose of it properly. A washable sticky mat is also available for this purpose from cleanroom supply companies.

VERIFYING OPERATIONAL CONDITIONS

When the operator and supplies have been prepared for introduction into the buffer zone, verification of proper operation of all equipment and engineering controls should be performed and documented. This may include checking and recording the operating pressure of the cleanroom complex, refrigerator and freezer temperatures, and hood performance and cleaning. It may also include verification that scheduled housekeeping has been performed, as well as cleaning and calibration of automated compounding devices, pumps, and other equipment. The certification sticker on the hoods should be checked to assure that performance testing is current. The operator should also verify proper operation by checking magnihelic gauges, or airflow displays.

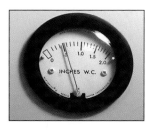

The magnihelic gauge on the front of some hoods indicates the pressure in the plenum area. Ask the service technician who tests your hood to indicate the proper operating range on the gauge, and verify this value each time you use the hood. Changes in the magnihelic are an indication that the

Figure 15. Magnihelic Gauge.

hood is no longer operating properly. A radical shift in the operating pressure may indicate that the motor/blower system is not operating properly, that HEPA filters are loaded, or that blockage of airflow has occurred. However, velocities may gradually shift outside the specified operating range without registering a significant change in the magnihelic reading. Also, unseen damage to HEPA filters which will result in leakage can easily occur. Routine, periodic testing must be carried out to confirm proper operation[8].

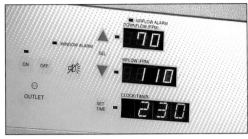

Some modern hood designs incorporate a probe which measures the actual velocities within the cabinet. Have the service technician indicate the proper operating ranges on the certification sticker, and verify proper performance each time you use the hood. This type of hood should sound an alarm if performance is out of range, also.

Figure 16. Air Inflow and downflow velocity display.

Any out-of-limits conditions must be reported immediately to supervisory personnel. Corrective action **must be performed prior to compounding,** or the entire process may be compromised. There is no point in validating a processing system if compounding is then performed when validation conditions have been compromised.

Objective 4.2) Prepare hoods for aseptic compounding.

Key Concept: Laminar Airflow hoods provide <u>only</u> a wash of clean air and work surfaces that are easy to clean and disinfect. When activities are preformed in the hood, contaminants are introduced to the work surface and can be transferred to product. Hoods must therefore be effectively cleaned and disinfected prior to each use. No matter how they look, you have no way of knowing or proving they have not become contaminated since their last use.

ESTABLISHING THE ASEPTIC FIELD FOR CRITICAL COMPOUNDING

The following procedures should be used to prepare the hood for compounding:

General Directions For All Laminar Flow Equipment

1. If the hood has been turned off, allow it to run for 15 to 30 minutes prior to use, to purge downstream contamination from HEPA filter surfaces.

2. All unnecessary items should be removed from the hood (this should be done at the end of each compounding procedure). Debris in the hood is a possible source of several types of contamination, and unnecessary items crowd and clutter the work space.

3. The hood should be cleaned with a **water-based, low-residue cleaner** (high pH for antineoplastic agents) at the start and end of each shift, whenever residue or debris accumulate, and between each compounding batch. This helps reduce **cross-contamination**. Alcohol disinfection alone may not remove all drug residues because not all substances are alcohol-soluble. Bleach or other heavily chlorinated solutions are not recommended for stainless steel surfaces, because they may cause pitting, making it difficult or impossible to completely clean the surface. Laminar airflow equipment disinfectant products validated for this application are available. Low-particulating, disposable wipes should be used. Cleaning materials used in a BSC where hazardous substances are compounded should be disposed of as hazardous waste.

4. Never attempt to clean a HEPA filter.

Alcohol Disinfection

Although 70% alcohol is a disinfectant, it is **not a sterilant.** If used properly, alcohol does kill many (but not all) vegetative organisms, and can decrease the bioburden in the hood and on other surfaces, such as gloves, bottles, and vials, thus reducing the probability of contamination. Items wiped or sprayed with alcohol are <u>not</u> **sterile,** but are only bacteriostatic. **Proper manipulative technique must be employed.**

Alcohol kills organisms by dehydration of the cells. To be effective, it must first penetrate the cell in a sufficient quantity to cause dehydration severe enough to kill the cell. This is known as **plasmolysis.** The alcohol must then be allowed to dry, since this is when the fatal dehydration occurs. **Low concentration** alcohols may not cause sufficient dehydration to kill cells due to **insufficient concentration,** while **high concentration** alcohols have **insufficient "dwell-time"** and may evaporate too quickly to penetrate microorganisms, many of which form protective coatings or spores. Because 70% alcohol has the optimum balance of these two qualities, it is the only concentration of alcohol that should be used for disinfection.

Alcohol must dry to be effective. If microorganisms become suspended in alcohol on the vial closures, they may be picked up on the needle as it penetrates the septum. Once introduced into the drug solution, the alcohol may become too diluted with drug solution to kill microorganisms. Thus, alcohol not allowed to dry properly may become a vehicle for the transfer of contaminants to the product. Also, alcohol may be an undesirable cross-contaminant in drug products, and must dry before compounding procedures commence for this reason, as well.

Because alcohol solutions may become contaminated, it is recommended that all bottles be discarded when empty, and not be reused. Sanitize the spray head with disinfectant before transferring to a new container.

CLEANING THE LAMINAR FLOW CLEAN BENCH (LFCB)

Using a water-based, high pH, disinfectant cleaner, followed by 70% alcohol, cleaning of an LFCB should be performed using a method which prevents dripping of dirty solution onto cleaned surfaces, and which does not carry contaminants from surfaces near the open end of the hood to the rear.

1. **In an HFCB, clean the top** of the hood, wiping in side-to-side, overlapping strokes, and working outward, from back to front. **In a VFCB, start at the top of the back,** moving parallel to the top of the cabinet, and work downward toward the worksurface. Clean the **IV pole and all hooks.**

2. Clean the **sides of the hood,** wiping from top to bottom, working outward from rear to front. In a VFCB, clean the **inside and outside** of the sash.

3. Clean the **work surface,** again wiping in side-to-side, overlapping strokes, working outward from rear to front.

4. **Disinfect the hood by spraying with 70% IPA, and allow to dry.**

CLEANING THE BIOLOGICAL SAFETY CABINET (BSC)

Cleaning of BSCs should be performed as follows:

1. **Gown as described for compounding hazardous substances,** but wear **three pair of gloves;** one inner pair, under the cuff of the gown, and two, heavy-weight, disposable pairs over the cuff.

2. Stage the following items:

    a. **A sealable chemo-waste container** small enough to fit in the hood, but large enough to accommodate cleaning waste,

    b. a **chemo disposal bag** large enough to contain the waste container,

c. **two chemo-resistant mats** (or one mat cut in half),

d. **one additional pair of outer gloves,**

e. at least **10 low-linting, disposable wipes,**

f. a high pH, low-residuing, **water-based cleaner** (many hazardous compounds are polar molecules, and are not soluble in alcohol, which is non-polar), and,

g. **70% IPA** for final disinfection.

A large chemo disposal container should be available immediately outside the BSC.

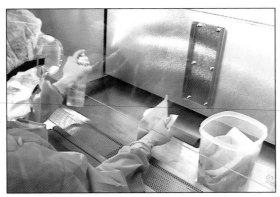

Figure 17. Keep one hand clean for spraying. Use the other for wiping.

3. While working, keep one hand clean, and do not set cleaner or alcohol containers in the hood, or any item directly on an uncleaned surface of the hood. Use the other hand for cleaning. **DO NOT open the sash above the marked operating height.** This practice reduces the velocity of protective inflowing air.

4. Place a chemo mat on the work surface and set the waste container upon it. **Using the clean hand, spray** cleaner on the front lip and front grill of the cabinet. **Using the other hand, clean** the lip first, starting at the bottom, working inward, and across the top of the front grill. Dispose of the wipe in the chemo container. This is done first to minimize transfer of contaminants to the gown sleeves.

5. Again, using the clean hand to apply cleaner and the dirty hand to wipe, clean the back of the hood, working from top to bottom.

6. Following the same procedure, clean **the IV pole,** then **the sides of the BSC,** and finally **the work surface** of the hood, using the same cleaning pattern as in the VFCB. After the entire work surface has been cleaned (except the area where the chemo mat and waste container are sitting) **transfer the waste container to the cleaned surface,** then **pick up the mat** by pinching it near the middle, in order that the dirty underside is folded to the inside, and dispose of in the waste container.

7. **Finish cleaning the work surface** and the **inside of the view screen.** Move the container to the front grill and lift the work surface. Place the second chemo mat in the undertray area and transfer the container to the mat. Now **prop the work surface against the back of the cabinet,** underside facing forward. Do not remove the grills and work surface from the hood.

8. Because the clean hand was used to manipulate the work surface, it may be contaminated. **Change the outer pair of gloves,** and, maintaining cleanliness of the spraying hand, **clean the underside of the work surface.**

9. Next, **turn over the front grill, clean the back,** and prop it against the work surface. **Now clean the undertray.** The undertray areas may contain sharp edges. Use care to avoid snagging or cutting your gloves. **Do not allow alcohol swabs, paper towels, labels, etc. to be drawn up into the plenum of the hood.** Such items may cause damage to the hood, but can only be removed by professionals trained to open the contaminated plenum of the hood safely. Newer hoods have a paper catch to prevent items from being drawn up which **must be routinely cleared of debris to prevent blockage of airflow.**

10. When all of the undertray except the area on which the mat and container are sitting has been cleaned, **move the container to a clean surface, dispose of the mat** as described in step 6, and **clean the remainder of the undertray.** Remove the outermost pair of gloves, and dispose of in the container. Seal the container, place in the bag (there is some possibility that the outer surfaces of the container have become contaminated). Seal the bag and transfer to the chemo container outside the hood.

11. **Spray the undertray area, back of the grill and work surface with IPA,** and return them to their original positions. **Spray all upper surfaces** of the hood with IPA and place a new chemo container in the hood. Remove the second pair of outer gloves, and dispose of them in the container. Clean the outside of the view screen.

12. De-gown properly and dispose of in the chemo container outside the hood.

Objective 4.3) Stage materials for compounding in the hood correctly.

Key Concept: Materials should be staged prior to compounding in order that introduction of contaminants into the work space is minimized, and to ensure that the correct components are used.

ANALYZE THE RISK FACTORS AND PLAN THE PROCESS DURING STAGING

Staging is the time when the compounding procedure should be planned, step-by-step. In a manufacturing environment, every step of a process is defined in a written procedure which must be followed exactly. Because IV admixtures compounding is extemporaneous, each compounding procedure is slightly different. Although there are general operational rules for specific types of compounding, the operator must **evaluate the tasks** at hand, determining which **core techniques** are required, the proper **order of manipulations,** and **all tools and components** required to complete the process.

Careful planning will minimize the number of reentries into the hood, and improve mental focus and accuracy. The compounding plan should be based on the physicians order, which must be read carefully. Be sure to identify the method of administration, and stage all materials required to accommodate it. Special procedures are usually employed for intrathecal preparations, and are required for hazardous compounds.

It is recommended that the component name, concentration, and amount required be quietly read aloud from the label or order. This improves recognition of the additives, and imprints them more effectively in the short-term memory. If the additive labels are also read aloud in the same manner, the chance of error will be greatly reduced. This also allows other personnel to hear, and mentally check, the accuracy of your interpretation of the order.

Staging should be conducted in the following manner:

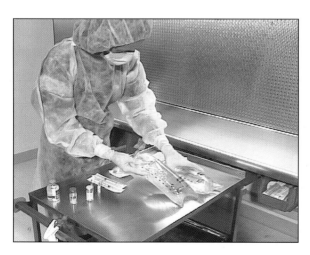

1. All outer wrappers not required to maintain sterility should be removed prior to introduction of supplies into the work area. Items for **one batch only** should be placed on a cleaned and disinfected cart or tray. All materials required for the batch

Figure 18. Stage and check all working materials prior to introduction to the work zone to assure accuracy and purity.

PART FOUR: ASEPTIC MANIPULATIONS

should be staged, including final containers, syringes, filter needles, transfer sets, diluents and drugs, seals, labels, etc.

2. All components to be used should be checked for proper identity, concentration, expiration date, container integrity, color, clarity, and particulates (in the case of solutions) to assure that the correct drug and dose are delivered. This check should be carried out with frequent reference to the order. All calculations should be made and cross-checked. When using previously-opened bulk containers, verify proper storage and check all required information on the ID label. **DO NOT use improperly stored vials, or vials with incomplete ID labels.**

3. All components should be wiped free of dust and dirt, and disinfected prior to introduction into the hood.

4. When compounding hazardous materials, the operator should assure that the **Material Safety Data Sheet (MSDS)** for the drug compounded is available for emergency personnel. Safety and emergency room personnel are not necessarily familiar with chemotherapeutic agents compounded in pharmacy and may need access to the Material Safety Data Sheet. The operator must read the MSDS and understand the proper emergency handling of the drug. A copy of the spill and exposure policies and procedures should also be available, and the operator must be completely familiar with these policies and procedures. Any chemo spill kits, eye wash stations, warning signs, or other equipment and materials required by policy must be available.

Objective 4.4) Properly arrange materials in the work space.

Key Concept: All critical sites must be placed so that they are constantly in "first air" after disinfection. Proper arrangement of materials in the work space reduces the risk of contamination and the risk of confusion and errors when compounding.

ARRANGEMENT OF MATERIALS IN A HORIZONTAL FLOW HOOD

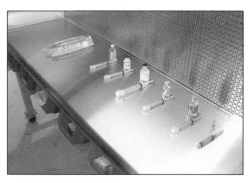

1. Components should be placed at one side of the work space, but at least three inches from the side of the hood, or any large equipment, and at least six inches in from the front opening of the hood.

Figure 19. Proper arrangement of materials in an LFCB

2. Components should be arranged in a single line, parallel to, and near the HEPA filter. They should be placed in such a way that injection ports or other critical surfaces are in the flow of first air.

3. A work space, not directly over the components, should be left open, so that manipulations can be carried out without working over disinfected critical sites. This work space should be at least six inches in from the front, and three inches from the sides of the hood.

4. Finished product should be placed at one side of the work space, to be removed when the batch is completed. Debris should also be placed at the side of the work space, but separate from product, preferably near the side of the hood on a tray.

5. Paper products should be kept out of the hood, except when they are necessary to maintain sterility (e.g. syringe and needle wrappers). It may, however, be desirable to have the label or order in view while compounding. It may be placed near the front and towards the end of the hood, well away from components and the work space. For hazardous materials, a plastic bag should be used to prevent label contamination.

ARRANGEMENT OF MATERIALS IN A VERTICAL FLOW HOOD

1. Components should be placed at one side of the work space, but at least three inches from the side of the hood, or any large equipment, and at least six inches in from the front opening.

2. Components should be arranged so that **first air, coming from above the work surface is supplied to all critical sites.** A "checkerboard" pattern may be used but care must be taken not to obstruct the first air with hands or objects. The ports of bags hanging from an IV pole in a VFCB are <u>not</u> located in first air. It is acceptable to attach a repeating syringe or transfer set to a bag aseptically, and then hang it from the pole, but care must be taken when returning the syringe to the hook to avoid puncturing the HEPA filter just above it.

3. Other aspects of compounding are conducted in a manner similar to that used in HFCBs.

ARRANGEMENT OF MATERIALS IN A BIOLOGICAL SAFETY CABINET

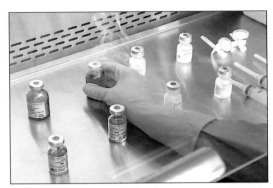

Figure 20. Smoke pattern showing proper arrangement of materials in a BSC.

1. Components should be placed at one side of the work space, but at least three inches from the side of the hood, or any large equipment, and at least three inches behind the front grill.

2. As in the VFCB, components should be arranged so that first air, coming from above the work surface is supplied to all critical sites, and is never obstructed by hands or objects. Avoid placing critical sites or working directly under the smoke-split.

As the unidirectional-flowing air approaches the worksurface, a **zone of confusion** is created, and it is necessary to be sure that critical sites remain in "first air". Also, the ports of bags hanging from an IV pole in a BSC are <u>not</u> located in first air, and care must be exercised to avoid damaging the HEPA filter above the work zone. Note: There is also an exhaust HEPA filter at the top of a BSC which can be damaged if items are placed on the top of the hood.

3. A work space, not directly over the components, should be left open, so that manipulations can be carried out without working directly over disinfected critical sites. This work space should be at least three inches behind the front grill of the hood.

4. Finished product should be placed at one side of the work space, to be removed when the unit or batch is completed. Debris should be placed on the other side of the work space, separate from product, preferably in a puncture-resistant, sealable container, labeled properly. All liquids should be in closed systems, and likewise placed in such a container, along with any other potentially contaminated items. Syringe wrappers, swab wrappers, etc., if not overtly contaminated, can be placed in a sealable plastic bag for transfer to a puncture-proof container outside the hood. These containers should be clearly marked with appropriate hazardous substance labels[14].

5. **Under no circumstances should any item whatsoever be placed on or against the grills of the hood.** This practice disrupts the normal airflow patterns of the hood and may compromise sterility, containment, or both by preventing the capture of inflowing and outflowing air.

6. General compounding activities should not be carried out in a BSC which is dedicated to hazardous materials compounding. Cross-contamination of these drugs may easily occur.

After arranging materials in the hood, remove any flip-top caps and disinfect all critical sites by spraying or swabbing with alcohol. Alcohol swabs should be used only once. **While the alcohol is drying, mentally work through the process again and select syringes, dispensing pins, filter needles, caps, and other tools that will be required to complete the compounding process.** Be aware of drug products or administration protocols which require special procedures and/or tools. Follow your institution's protocol for all such situations.

Stage compounding tools in the hood near the staged components and final containers. Disinfect gloves and allow them to dry in the laminar airflow slipstream. This is a good time to have a pharmacist verify that the proper components have been selected, and to reread the order and component labels. Compounding activities may commence when the alcohol has dried, and pharmacist approval obtained. **Redisinfect gloves each time you leave and re-enter the aseptic field.**

Objective 4.5) Select the appropriate compounding tools for each task.

Key Concept: The proper tools must be used to accomplish the desired product quality. To select the proper tools, you must understand the design of each tool, and its appropriate use.

NEEDLES: A needle consists of two parts; the needle shaft (cannula) and the hub. The hollow bore of the needle shaft is called the lumen. The hub is the portion to which a syringe attaches. The needle cap should be kept on until the time of use and should then be removed so that the shaft is in first air.

Needle size is designated by length and gauge. The length of a needle is measured in inches from the juncture of the hub and the shaft to the tip of the point, and ranges from three-eighths to three and one-half inches, or longer. Needles should be long enough to penetrate well into the final bag to assure adequate mixing.

The gauge of a needle is a measure of the outside diameter of the shaft, and ranges from 29, the finest, to 13, the largest. **The finer the needle, the higher the gauge number.** The choice of the needle size is determined mainly by the viscosity of the drug solution, and the nature of the closures to be penetrated. The highest possible gauge needles are desirable, since they are less likely to leave an unsealed hole in the closure. This is especially true when multiple entries will be made through a sep-

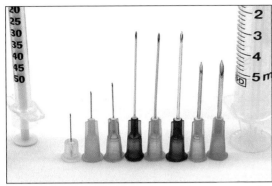

Figure 21. Needles arranged from higher gauge on the left, to lower gauge on the right.

tum, or when compounding hazardous substances. Avoid re-entering an existing needle hole, because this tends to enlarge the hole and increases the potential for leakage and coring. Thicker (smaller gauge) needles may be needed for more viscous solutions.

Filter needles and filter straws are used to remove bits of debris and particulates from solutions. **The contents of ampules should always be filtered,** because bits of glass and other debris may fall into the neck when the ampule is opened. Filtration should be in one direction, only. It is usually easier to push fluids through a filter than to draw them up, however, syringes to be sent to the floor must be filtered when they are drawn.

SYRINGES: The two basic parts of a syringe are the **barrel** and the **plunger.** The barrel is a tube which is open at one end to allow insertion of the plunger, with a hollow hub at the other end for needle attachment. The open end has flanges to prevent the barrel from slipping through the fingers during manipulation. The plunger is a cone-shaped, piston-like tip, operated by a rod (shaft) which passes inside the barrel. The other end of the plunger is a flat thrust surface (disk, or "button") for easy manipulation. Because the shaft of the plunger can carry contaminants into the barrel of the syringe, it should not be touched in a way that can lead to contamination. This is called **"palming the plunger"**. If it is necessary to handle the shaft of the plunger when handling particularly awkward containers or hazardous materials to avoid the risk of contamination of product or exposure to hazardous substances, **the syringe <u>must</u> <u>not</u> be reused.** Do not make excessive adjustments of the plunger which might carry contaminants to the portion of the barrel containing product, and do not reuse the syringe. **(Syringe reuse is never recommended)**

Syringes should be **large enough to accommodate the required volume and allow space** for removing bubbles and adjusting the final volume, but small enough to ensure accuracy. **The dose to be drawn should be at least 20% of the capacity of the syringe.** When compounding hazardous substances, the syringe should never be more than 3/4 full.

The hub of the syringe barrel provides the point of attachment for a needle. The tip may be tapered to allow the needle hub to be slipped over it with a twisting motion, and held on by friction ("interference fit"). When this method is used, the needle is reasonably secure, but it may slip off the tip of the syringe under some circumstances. Remove all needle caps by pulling straight outward without twisting. Most syringes currently used in pharmacy have a "luer" tip. **All syringes and syringe caps used for hazardous materials should have Luer-lok™ type connections in which the needle twists into a special locking groove.** The volume of solution inside a syringe is indicated by the graduation lines on the barrel. **Do not assume that a vial or ampule contains the exact dosage indicated on the label.** Use the graduations on the syringe to measure the dose accurately.

Special-purpose syringes, such as tuberculin and insulin syringes are graduated in special ways. Tuberculin syringes have a total capacity of one milliliter, and their long, slender, barrels allow for more precise graduation scales. Insulin syringes are graduated in both milliliters and insulin units. When working with small-dose syringes, special procedures must be used if needles are to be changed, because the needle may retain a significant percentage of the dose measured. If needles must be changed, draw up an excess of the product and adjust the final measurement **after** the needle has been changed and the new needle is refilled.

Reuse of syringes, needles, and other disposable tools is not recommended. Needles dull quickly, which increases the chance of coring rubber or plastic septa. Reuse also increases the potential for microbiologic and cross-contamination. **The same syringe should never be used for two different drug products, even if they are going into the same admixture.** First, the vial from which drug is drawn may become cross-contaminated. Also, certain drug products are incompatible in their concentrated form, and may cause precipitation if they come into contact before they have been diluted in the final solution.

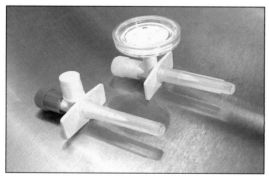

Figure 22. Dispensing pins may have "<u>hydrophobic</u>" filters for hazardous substances (upper), or "<u>hydrophilic</u>" filters for general use. (lower)

DISPENSING PINS: There are several types of dispensing devices (or "pins") available for multi-dose vials. These devices are vented through air filters which allow vial pressure to equalize and prevent the introduction of contaminants. Devices with **hydrophilic filters** are acceptable for routine compounding. However, when compounding hazardous substances, only **hydrophobic filters,** which do not allow droplets of liquid to pass through them under pressure, are acceptable. Dispensing devices have thick spikes, which punch a large hole in the rubber closure. Therefore, they should not be removed, once inserted.

Objective 4.6) Evaluate risk factors, correctly perform core manipulative techniques used for various component packaging systems and devices, and understand the methods to be used in developing compounding procedures.

Key Concept: A precise method of performing manipulations should be learned and followed exactly, so that good aseptic technique becomes habit. An evaluation of the particular contamination risks in a given process will be valuable in developing correct procedures, keeping in mind the design of the engineering controls you employ, and the barrier controls you wear.

We will present a number of "**core**" techniques, which are fundamental to processes, pointing out the particular risks to be considered in each technique. We will also present several commonly-encountered packaging systems. When new tools or processes are encountered, techniques and procedures should be developed, written, validated, and practiced by all personnel.

ASSEMBLING A NEEDLE AND SYRINGE: RISK FACTORS:

1. Touch contamination of exposed syringe and needle hubs.

2. Airborne contamination due to disruption of first air to critical sites and pathways.

PROCEDURE:

Paper-wrapped syringes with hub covers should be removed from the wrapper when they are placed in the hood. **Syringes** without hub covers **must be assembled with the needle immediately upon opening or should be left in the** 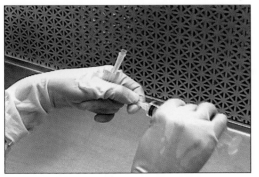 **wrapper until time of use.** When using syringes with hub covers and paper wrapped needles, opening the needle requires the most dexterity in the assembly process. Therefore, begin by grasping the flaps of the paper needle cover and pull them back, folding them down along the

Figure 23. Grasp the needle between the last three fingers and the palm, freeing the thumb and forefinger for manipulation of the syringe hub cover.

sides of the needle with the open hub of the needle pointed into first air. Keeping fingers well away from the exposed hub of the needle, lodge the needle tip securely between the palm and the last three fingers. Pick up the syringe with the other hand and, using the thumb and forefinger of the needle hand, twist the cap off the syringe. Bring the needle and syringe together in first air, and secure the needle to the syringe by twisting gently to activate the lock (See Fig. 23).

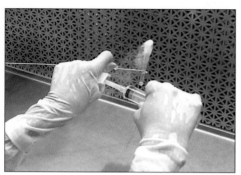

Figure 24. Maintain a clear path for first air to flow over the needle/syringe junction.

For syringes **without hub covers,** or those contained in plastic housings, opening the syringe requires the most dexterity. Start by picking up the syringe and remove the packaging, making sure the exposed hub tip is maintained in first air. While holding the syringe with the last three fingers and palm, proceed with opening the needle as described previously, using the thumb and index finger of the syringe hand and the free hand to open the needle.

For **needles with plastic hubs covers**, prepare the syringe, then hold the needle in the opposite hand and use the thumb and the forefinger of the syringe hand to remove the needle hub cover. Bring the needle and syringe together in first air, and secure the needle to the syringe by twisting gently to activate the lock. The practice of "popping' the needle hub through the needle wrapper exposes the inside of the needle to particulates released when the paper tears. **This can result in both particulate and microbial contamination because the outside of the needle wrapper in not sterile.** Minimize the amount of time that needles, spikes, and unprotected hubs as critical pathways are exposed by pre-planning all operations and pre-assembling the materials required for each step. Opened needles and syringes should be assembled immediately and needle caps should not be removed until use.

CHANGING NEEDLES

Although "Universal Precautions" for blood-borne pathogens forbid the recapping of needles following administration to the patient, it is sometimes necessary in pharmacy to recap needles in order to remove the needle, and change to a cap, filter needle or straw. There is no blood-borne hazard to the operator during IV compounding, and the needle remains sterile, posing no infection hazard. However, extreme caution must still be exercised to avoid accidental skin punctures. Needle recapping during hazardous materials compounding requires careful technique because a puncture can also constitute an exposure hazard and should be avoided.

ENTERING A VIAL: RISK FACTORS:

1. Touch contamination.

2. Airborne contamination due to disruption of first air.

3. Contaminant transfer from septa and other surfaces.

4. Particulate contamination due to "coring".

PROCEDURE:

The rubber-type septum through which the needle enters a vial or bottle is a critical site. It should be free of dirt and debris, disinfected with 70% alcohol and allowed to dry completely. Alcohol may be supplied either on individually-wrapped swabs, or in spray bottles. If swabs are used, they should be used only once, because they tend to dry out quickly and may not deliver a sufficient amount of alcohol to more than one injection site to kill microorganisms. They may also transfer contaminants, lint and other debris from one critical site to another. Manipulate vials and bottles so that the supply of first air to the septum is never interrupted. Avoid working above disinfected septa and opening syringe and needle wrappers in a way that may cause particles to fly toward the septa.

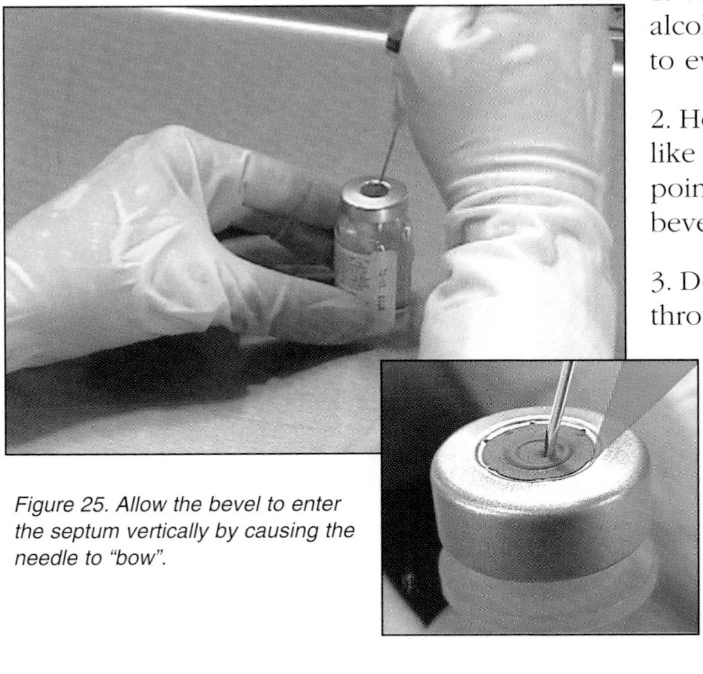

Figure 25. Allow the bevel to enter the septum vertically by causing the needle to "bow".

1. Wipe the stopper with an alcohol swab or spray and allow to evaporate.

2. Hold the syringe in one hand like a pencil with the needle pointing down and allow the bevel point to touch the septum.

3. Do not force the needle through the septum. Rather, as the needle begins to penetrate the septum apply slight lateral pressure to the syringe so the needle shaft bends slightly, in the direction opposite from the bevel. This will cause the needle to **"bow"** slightly, and the bevel to

become perpendicular to the septum. Bowing the needle is done to reduce the incidence of "coring", especially with large gauge needles, short bevels, and multiple needle entries.

FILLING THE SYRINGE FROM A VIAL: RISK FACTORS:

1. Touch contamination.

2. Airborne contamination due to disruption of first air.

3. Contaminant transfer from septa and other surfaces.

4. Particulate contamination due to "coring".

5. Exposure of operator or environmental contamination due to drug release.

6. Incorrect dosing due to inaccurate measurement.

7. Incorrect dosing due to improperly stored drug in multiple-use vials.

PROCEDURE:

1. Select the additive or diluent required by the order. Assure that it is the correct drug, has the correct concentration, and is not expired. If using a stored, reusable vial, assure that the drug was properly stored, and that all required information is on the pharmacy identification label affixed to the vial, including date of opening, pharmacy use expiration date, and operator initials. For reconstituted product the diluent used and final concentration must also be included. **If any of this information is not supplied, it is not possible to know the concentration and potency of the product, and it cannot be used.** Check all containers for integrity, solution color and clarity, precipitate and particulates.

2. Wipe the septum with an alcohol swab or spray with alcohol, and allow to evaporate.

The "**low-pressure**" (see-saw) technique is recommended for all compounding activities and required for compounding of hazardous substances. Spray produced when pressure builds up in a vial may escape from the vial or the syringe when they are separated and overcome the protective air curtain in a BSC, and spray also introduces undesirable cross-contaminants and filth in the work zone of any hood.

3. **Do not** draw up a volume of air equal to the volume of fluid to be removed from the vial. Rather, draw up a volume of air 5 to 10 mL less than the volume

of liquid to be withdrawn. As you gain experience, you will become familiar with the proper amounts for each situation. Insert the needle into the vial septum without coring.

4. Lift the vial with inserted needle and syringe from the counter top and invert them as one unit, maintaining first air to the needle/septum junction at all times.

The inverted vial may be wedged between the first two fingers, held as you would make a "V" sign. Hold the barrel of the syringe between the remaining two fingers and the thumb, leaving the opposite hand free to operate the plunger. For larger

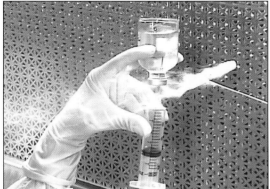

vials, grasp the base of the vial with one hand, maintaining "first air" flow to the critical needle/septum junction. The other hand is used to grasp the button of the plunger. To manipulate the plunger, place the forefinger of this hand against the flange of the syringe barrel and press against it.

Figure 26. The "V" grip can be used to control the vial and syringe with one hand while maintaining first air flow as demonstrated by smoke.

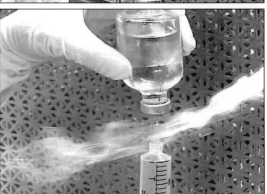

Figure 27. Maintain "first air" flow in an HFCB as illustrated by smoke.

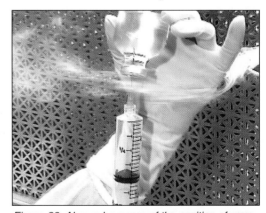

Figure 28. Always be aware of the position of your hands and fingers relative to the flow of first air. Do not block first air, as shown above.

In a Biological Safety Cabinet, or a Vertical Flow Cleanbench, the flow of first air is best maintained by holding the vial and syringe in a more horizontal position, with the vial elevated above the syringe. (See figure 29)

5. Keep the inverted vial in place between the fingers, and rotate the barrel of the syringe so that the graduated measurement scale can be read.

6. **DO NOT PUSH AIR INTO THE VIAL AGAINST PRESSURE.** Gradually pull back on the plunger to draw fluid into the syringe barrel, keeping the needle point below the fluid surface at all times. As fluid is withdrawn, a partial vacuum is created in the vial. As the vacuum becomes difficult to overcome, release the plunger so that the vacuum will cause air to be drawn into the vial from the syringe, assisting slightly as necessary. Repeat this process in a **"see-saw"** fashion as required to draw up the desired dose. Keep the bevel in the fluid as the level of the fluid declines.

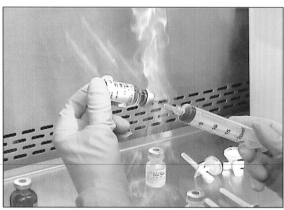

Figure 29. Smoke demonstrating flow of first air in a BSC.

7. Gently tap the outside of the barrel to free any air bubbles, and make the final volume adjustment.

8. Remove the vial from the needle. You will hear a slight hiss, as air rushes equally into the vial and needle tip. This process prevents squirting and splattering of drug. Have a pharmacist check the plunger position. With the needle pointed up in first air, draw up sufficient air into the needle to clear the fluid from the shaft if the needle is to be removed. Do not push air and residual drug in the needle out into the hood.

RECONSTITUTING A VIAL: RISK FACTORS:

1. Touch contamination.

2. Airborne contamination due to disruption of first air.

3. Contaminant transfer from septa and other surfaces.

4. Particulate contamination due to "coring".

5. Exposure of operator or environmental contamination due to drug release.

6. Incorrect dosing due to inaccurate measurement.

7. Incorrect dosing due to incomplete dissolution of drug or mixing of the solution.

PROCEDURE:

1. Verify that the drug and diluent are correct and acceptable for use. Disinfect the stopper and maintain in first air.

2. Fill a syringe with diluent as described above. Insert the biased needle bevel into the septum of the drug vial, bowing to prevent coring, and pull back on the plunger, creating negative pressure in the vial by removing air from the vial into the syringe. **Do Not Push Fluid** into the vial against pressure. Allow diluent to flow into the vial, assisting by pushing the plunger gently, but not beyond its starting point. When diluent stops flowing easily, draw back on the plunger again and repeat the process using "**See-Saw**" technique, until all diluent has been transferred to the vial.

3. Gently swirl the vial/syringe assembly in first air until all drug is dissolved. If the drug is to be drawn up immediately, the syringe may be left upright in the vial and placed in first air, near the HEPA filter. To swirl, secure the barrel of the syringe with the first two fingers and the vial with the last two fingers and thumb. Maintain first air flow and swirl the assembly to dissolve.

4. Check reconstituted drug vials for complete dissolution, color, clarity, and particulates. Re-disinfect the vial septum before using further.

5. Apply a pharmacy identification label to the vial, and store according to label or insert instructions and your institution's policies. Include date and time of reconstitution, pharmacy use expiration, diluent name and amount, final concentration and initials.

USE OF AMPULES: RISK FACTORS:

1. Touch contamination.

2. Ampules present an **increased risk of particulate contamination** because debris on the neck and fragments of glass may fall into it when it is opened.

3. Ampules present an **increased risk of airborne contamination** due to the large, open pathway created when the top is removed.

4. Ampules present an **increased risk of injury to the operator, or damage** to the HEPA filter due to flying fragments of glass when they are opened.

5. Ampules present an **increased risk of exposure to drug product** for the operator and environment due to the splattering of drug remaining in the top or coating the inner surface of the neck.

PROCEDURE:

Opening an Ampule

Because the open neck of the ampule provides a large pathway for the entrance of contaminants, all contents should be drawn up immediately upon opening. For this reason, **the syringe and needle should be prepared prior to opening the ampule. The unused portion of ampules must be discarded. Ampules cannot reliably be stored for later use, even in a laminar airflow hood.**

When an ampule is opened, fibers and particles of glass may fall inside. For this reason, **the neck of the ampule should be thoroughly cleaned with an alcohol swab,** disinfected prior to opening, and the **contents must be filtered prior to use.** The ampule should be snapped open towards the side of the hood to prevent glass fragments from damaging the HEPA filter or the operator. A sterile gauze pad should be wrapped around the neck of any ampules containing hazardous substances when they are opened to protect fingers and contain splatter, and may be used for all ampules to protect the fingers and minimize debris. **The use of alcohol pads for this purpose is not recommended, because alcohol may be expressed into the ampule, contaminating the product.**

The following steps should be followed each and every time an ampule is opened:

1. Check the label for content identity, concentration, and expiration date and the container for cracks and other signs of damage. Check for discoloration and visible particulate matter.

2. If fluid or powder is present in the stem, gently tap the sides of the ampule, or shake in a long, smooth stroke to remove material from the stem.

3. Wipe the neck of the ampule with an alcohol swab to clean and wipe with a fresh swab or spray with alcohol to disinfect. Allow to dry.

4. Be sure the syringe is assembled and ready to draw up the ampule contents immediately upon opening.

5. Place the thumb on the top, near the neck on the side nearest you with the opposite side facing the side of the hood, and pinch the stem between the thumb and forefinger, making certain it is secure. Some ampules are marked with a dot to indicate proper placement of the thumb. Place the thumb of the other hand similarly just below the neck and grasp the body of the ampule. **DO NOT POINT the ampule directly toward the HEPA filter.** It should be broken open toward the side panels which will minimize the chance of glass chips

or small amounts of the contents flying into the filter. Snap the stem off by pushing with the thumbs while pulling back with the other fingers, gently but persistently, until the ampule "pops" open.

6. Immediately draw up the contents of the ampule, and discard any unused contents as contaminated waste. The ampule and top should be discarded in a sharps container. In the case of ampules used for hazardous materials, any remaining fluid must be disposed of in a closed system.

7. Filter the contents of the ampule.

Filling The Syringe From an Ampule

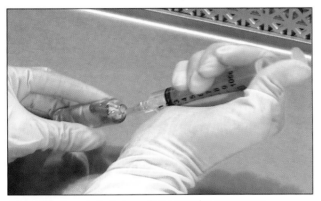

Figure 30. Ampule technique demonstrating proper use of "first air".

1. Holding the ampule perpendicular to the first air flow and tilted slightly in one hand, and the syringe in the other, grasp the syringe with the palm up and the syringe lying across it in a manner that places the plunger button by the thumb, needle bevel down. Close the remaining fingers down over the barrel. The syringe hand should not be directly over the ampule.

2. Insert the tip of the needle into the neck of the opened ampule so that the bevel is facing downward just below the fluid level.

3. Place the thumb under the lip of the plunger button and extend it to draw up the fluid through the needle, as you move the ampule to a horizontal position, keeping the bevel submerged in the fluid.

4. When transferring a large volume into the syringe, the thumb may be too short to force the plunger far enough to draw up the desired volume. If this occurs, allow the syringe to slip down the hand a few centimeters, then reestablish your hand grip and continue extension of the plunger with your thumb. Draw up a slight excess above the required dose. Avoid pressing the needle against the bottom of the ampule or drawing up the last drops, because this fluid is most likely to contain glass fragments and other particulates.

5. Hold the syringe vertically, needle upward, and pull back slightly on the plunger to withdraw fluid from the needle. Replace the needle with a filter needle. Refill the filter needle and adjust to the final volume required, dripping the excess into a suitable container.

STORAGE OF UNUSED DRUG PRODUCT

1. Ampules are single-use containers and must not be reused. The open neck of the ampule is a clear pathway by which contaminants may readily enter the ampule.

2. For vials, <u>prior</u> to removing the vial from the hood, disinfect the rubber closure with alcohol. Tear a tamper-evident seal from the roll, leaving it intact on the paper backing until it is inside the hood. In first air, aseptically remove the seal from backing and apply directly to septum.

3. All vials should have an identification label (ID label) marked with the following information:

    a. The initials of person who opened/reconstituted the vial.

    b. Date and time of first use or reconstitution.

    c. Pharmacy use expiration date and time. Note any special storage requirements such as "protect from light", "refrigerate", or "do not refrigerate". Be certain the product is properly stored.

    d. The amount and name of the diluent added and final concentration for reconstituted products. It cannot be assumed that the standard dilution suggested on the label was used when the product was reconstituted, even if other identification information is marked. **Do not use reconstituted drug product that does not specify the amount and name of diluent used and the final concentration.**

If the vial label is small, or of slick paper that does not hold markings well, an auxiliary label should be used for the required information. If applying an auxiliary label, be careful not to cover other important information such as identity, concentration, or expiration date. If a vial is not clearly marked as required and properly stored, it should not be reused.

USE OF VENTED DISPENSING PINS: RISK FACTORS:

1. Use of dispensing pins presents an **increased risk of touch contamination** for two reasons:

a. Dispensing pin caps are frequently mishandled, which can lead to **contamination of multiple products.**

b. There are generally more manipulations involved in adding diluent to the product or withdrawing product for admixture to a final container because needles must be removed or attached, and the syringe must also be attached to, and removed from the pin. A larger number of manipulations presents a greater opportunity for contamination.

2. The risk of particulate contamination due to coring is **decreased.**

3. The risk of environmental contamination or operator exposure to drug is **decreased** if a pin with a *hydrophobic* filter is used properly. However, it is *increased* if a pin with a *hydrophilic* filter is used.

Other risk factors are similar to those already discussed.

PROCEDURE:

For vials with small septa, a thick pin may push the septum into the vial, rather than puncture it. Therefore, the use of dispensing pins is not recommended for vials with small closures. Also, not all drug can be removed with a dispensing pin due to the position of the pin inlet holes within the vial. **DO NOT** attempt to wiggle the pin back out when compounding hazardous materials in an attempt to extract more of the drug from the vial. Neither should pins be moved from one vial to another.

1. Disinfect the septum and allow to dry completely. Locate the vial so that the flow of first air over the septum will not be interrupted. Remove the spike cover by pulling straight out and insert into the middle of the septum.

2. If the contents are to be reconstituted, draw up the required volume of diluent in a syringe and recap the needle. As always, have a pharmacist verify the correct plunger position for proper volume, and the diluent name.

3. Remove the dispensing pin cap aseptically, and place it in first air, inside up.

4. Aseptically remove the syringe needle and twist the syringe onto the dispensing pin. Place the assembly on the worksurface and reconstitute as usual.

5. Aseptically remove the syringe and replace the dispensing pin cap.

6. Place a complete ID label on the vial.

7. When ready to withdraw the drug, aseptically remove the cap and place it in first air, inside up. Remove the hub cover or needle from a syringe and twist the syringe onto the dispensing pin hub.

8. Invert the assembly, keeping the critical sites in first air. Withdraw the required dose, remove any bubbles, and make the final dosage adjustment.

9. Turn the assembly to the horizontal position and carefully twist to unlock the connection between the syringe and dispensing pin, tipping both so that the open orifices are pointing upward and maintained in first air as they separate.

10. Set the vial aside in the first air and attach a needle or syringe cap to the syringe, as required. Aseptically replace the dispensing pin cap.

Dispensing pins must not be removed from the vial or be reused. **Care must also be taken to maintain the sterility of the dispensing pin cap.** It should be removed and replaced aseptically and maintained in first air when it is off. Careless handling of bulk containers and dispensing pin caps can lead to contamination of multiple containers. Vials **cannot** be stored in an LFCB or BSC without the dispensing pin cap in place.

USE OF REPEATING SYRINGES: RISK FACTORS:

1. Repeating syringes present an **increased** risk of **inaccurate measurement** if the device is not properly adjusted or if incorrect technique is used.

2. Repeating syringes present an **increased** risk of **cross-contamination** if needles are not changed.

3. The risk of touch contamination to the syringe can lead to contamination of multiple products.

Other risks are similar to those already discussed.

PROCEDURE:

1. If using a bag for the source solution, orient the administration port in first air and remove its plastic cover, taking care not to contaminate the sterile pathway. Remove the cap from the spike and insert it into the administration port, puncturing the inner seal. For unvented bottles, remove the metal cap and swab the stopper with alcohol. Insert the spike into the middle of the stopper. If a bottle with a vent tube is to be used, aseptically remove the metal cover and rubber seal. Insert the spike into the larger administration port, **not the vent tube.**

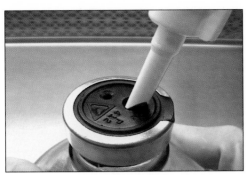

Figure 31. Be sure to insert spike in the large administration port site, not the vent tube hole.

2. Adjust the syringe to the desired dispensing volume by depressing the plunger to the desired volume, hold, and turn the retaining nut down the limiter rod to lock the plunger in place. Remove the syringe cap and aseptically attach a needle. Always use a vented needle or adapter to prevent build-up of pressure in the vial.

3. To prime the tubing and fill the syringe, depress the plunger completely, release and allow to return completely to the stop. Repeat this action until the tubing and syringe are completely filled. Replace the needle cap.

Before dispensing any fluid, have a pharmacist verify the correct fluid volume setting. Assume that the dispensing needle on any repeating syringe is used, and replace it prior to use. To assure the needle is uncontaminated, always change dispensing needles:

a. when you begin reconstitution,

b. when you begin reconstituting a different drug, and

c. at least every three to four uses, to minimize the chance of contamination and coring which is easily caused by dull needles.

When dispensing, always make sure the plunger is completely extended, and the barrel of the syringe is full. **Dispensing must be accomplished in a single, positive injection,** because allowing the plunger to rebound in "mid-stroke" will cause additional fluid to be be added into the syringe, changing the final volume delivered. Place a complete ID label on the reconstituted vial. **Do not use the same syringe and transfer set to dispense different fluids.**

INJECTING ADDITIVES INTO BAGS AND BOTTLES

It is useful to arrange all bags or bottles in a specific orientation or location at the start of operations (for example, with the additive port facing to the right for bags, or at one side of the work space for bottles), and turn or move each one in an exact way after additives have been injected, so that you can always tell which containers have been completed. It is not recommended that more than four containers with identical orders be staged at one time. **All containers in a hood at any one time must be for identical orders to avoid errors.**

All containers should be staged, and checked for container integrity, color, and precipitates. The label should be checked to verify identity, concentration and expiration date and the container prepared for introduction into the work zone as described. The hood should be cleaned and disinfected, and the operator properly attired and prepared. All additive ports must be disinfected and maintained in first air.

A pharmacist should verify plunger positions and cross-check all drug names, concentrations, volumes required, and expiration dates, as well as the final container diluent expiration date, identity, concentration, and volume against the order. The additives may then be injected into the bag or bottle.

INJECTING ADDITIVES INTO A PLASTIC BAG

The plastic bag is made of flexible polyvinyl chloride (PVC), or other specially formulated and approved plastic. Plastic bags are available in different sizes and have a flat extension with an eyelet to allow them to be hung on an administration pole. There are two main arrangements available in plastic bags. One has parallel additive and administration ports at the end, which are approximately the same length. The administration set port has a plastic cover. The additive port has a protective rubber septum. The other bag arrangement has the additive port located a quarter of the way up the bag on its front center ("belly-port").

The rubber septum on the additive port is self-sealing which prevents leaking of the solution from the port when punctured by a needle, however, repeated punctures of the rubber seal with an 18G or 19G needle will result in leakage from the port. To reduce this problem, special adaptors are available when multiple injections are required.

The plastic bag is a closed system and does not require outside air. Because of its flexibility, no vacuum is present in the plastic bag. When making additions to the plastic bag system, the admixtures specialist must exert pressure on the syringe plunger to introduce the additive to the solution.

Plastic bags are marked with graduations to indicate the approximate fluid volume in the bag, in both the upright and inverted positions. However, unlike their glass counterparts, stored plastic bags must be kept covered with a non-porous plastic outer bag. The outer bag will prevent the loss of fluid which would evaporate through the uncovered IV bag. The outer wrapper can be removed from the IV bag prior to use, but once removed, the contents of the inner bag should be used within 30 days, or as the manufacturer recommends.

Mix well after each addition, both to ensure uniformity of drug in the container, and to prevent any interactions or precipitation that might occur between additives if they are mixed in concentrated amounts, or in the wrong order. Add any incompatible substances first and last, with thorough mixing in between.

BAGS WITH END-TYPE ADDITIVE PORTS

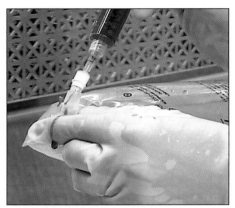

Figure 32. The needle may penetrate the back of the medication port tube, ruining the bag, and possibly causing injury.

When injecting into the additive port, be sure that fingers do not block the flow of first air. Approximately one-half inch inside each port, there is a diaphragm which must be punctured to enter the bag. The needle used to inject the bag must be long enough to puncture any inner seal in the tube portion of the additive port, and pass through the tube into the bag, so that additives will mix effectively. **Tuberculin or other short needles should not be used for injecting additives, because the drug may remain in the additive tube, below the diaphragm, preventing it from mixing with the diluent.** These syringes are often used to measure and add very small doses to an IV admixture. Therefore, the needle on a tuberculin syringe must be changed prior to drawing up a dose. This is done because the amount of fluid required to fill the new needle may be greater than the amount that was in the small tuberculin needle, and may represent a significant portion of the small dose normally drawn up in a tuberculin syringe.

Hold the medication port extended while adding drugs to assure proper insertion of the needle. Make sure to enter in a straight line so the needle does not puncture the wall of the additive tube. This will compromise sterility and can also result in a painful needle stick.

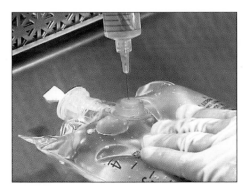

INJECTING ADDITIVES INTO A BAG WITH A "BELLY PORT"

Bags with the additive port on the face of the bag, known as a **"belly port"**, should be carefully sanitized prior to loading into the hood, especially all areas which remain upstream of

Figure 33. Maintain the port in first air, and use care to avoid puncturing the back of the bag.

the critical site. These bags cannot be maintained in first air when hanging from an IV pole, and should be placed on the work surface in a way which maximizes first air exposure. Care must be exercised to prevent a puncture of the rear side of the bag when injecting additives. This is accomplished by applying firm pressure on the upper half of the bag to distend the belly port area. Be sure to mix thoroughly after each addition.

INJECTING ADDITIVES INTO A BOTTLE

Solutions in glass bottles are packed under a vacuum and sealed by a rubber closure. Remove the aluminum disc, and swab or spray the stopper with alcohol. Allow to dry. The operator need only insert the syringe into the bottle, biasing the bevel of the needle to prevent coring and allow the contents of the syringe to be drawn in. The process can only be repeated a few times, because the vacuum is gradually lost. Swirl gently after each addition to mix completely.

Intravenous solution bottles are made of high-quality glass, and have molded graduation marks to show the approximate solution volume, both in the upright and inverted positions. Labels on solution bottles not only contain the usual descriptive and quality control information (expiration date/lot number) but also carry an inverted identification. The inverted information usually consists of only the name and concentration of the solution. When attaching a label to the finished admixture, do not cover up the inverted portion of the label, which will be upright when the bottle is attached to the administration pole. Also, do not place the label over the graduation marks on the bottle.

INJECTING ADDITIVES INTO A BOTTLE WITH A VENT TUBE

Bottles with vent tubes have a rubber disc under the metal cap, which covers the rubber stopper. The rubber stopper has three sites, two round perforations and a triangular site of less thickness than the rest of the rubber closure. The triangle-shaped site is intended for addition of supplemental medication while the admixture is being administered to the patient.

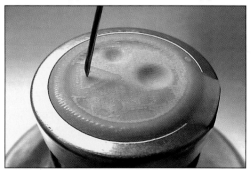

Figure 33. Inject additives into the triangle-shaped site.

The larger of the two perforations is an insert site for an administration set and the other is an opening to the air tube. The rubber disc which covers the sterile stopper is removed just prior to attachment of the administration set. Injection of additives is usually accomplished through the additive site, and rubber disc, with the vacuum intact. **Never inject additives into the vent tube.**

Bottles should be discarded if the vacuum is not intact when the aluminum cap is removed.

There are two ways to check if the vacuum is still intact:

a. A slight indentation of the rubber disc covering the air tube and administration openings should be visible.

b. An audible hiss should be heard when the rubber disc is removed for attachment of tubing (unless vacuum is neutralized by additives).

NEEDLE-LESS SYSTEMS

Several "needle-less" systems are available, and are intended to reduce the incidence of needle sticks. You should familiarize yourself with any systems in use in your institution. Aseptic technique must be used with needle-less systems, before, during, and after the cannula has been withdrawn from the stopper penetration spike. Some systems are not appropriate for hazardous substances because drug product remains on the outside of the spike when the cannula is withdrawn.

CONNECTING TUBING

When an IV administration set is to be attached in the pharmacy, it should be done prior to the addition of any drugs. Lay the bag laterally in first air, remove the plastic cover from the sterile administration port, taking care not to touch this port. Remove the cover from the administration set and discard. Key the administration spike in the port and push the spike firmly into the administration port, piercing the inner seal. For bottles with vent tubes, remove the latex disc, keeping the stopper in first air and immediately push the spike through the administration set site. For other bottles, swab or spray the stopper to disinfect, allow to dry, and push the administration set spike into the middle of the stopper.

Hang the bag or bottle and unfold the tubing. Aseptically place the delivery end in first air over a specimen cup or other receptacle and remove the set cover, setting it aside in first air. Open the flow regulator and slide clamps and prime the tubing. After priming, close the flow regulator and slide clamps, making sure they are secure. Re-cap the distal end of the tubing, carefully fold the tubing up, and secure it. Check that the tubing is secure and will not leak by pressing slightly on the bag to generate internal pressure while observing the closure for any leakage. Complete compounding as usual.

PREPARING SYRINGES

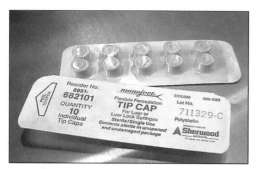

Figure 35. Push-on caps.

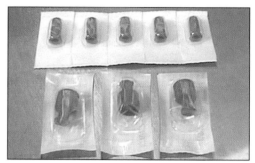

Figure 36. Twist-on caps should be used for hazardous substances.

When syringes are to be dispensed directly to the floors, the needle should normally be removed and replaced with a cap. Push-on caps often are provided in packages of 10, which may be opened to reveal 2 at a time, maintaining the sterility assurance seal to the remainder of the pack. The caps should be opened and placed in first air. When applying the cap, care should be taken to avoid contaminating the cap adjacent to it. Do not use caps left sitting open in the hood, because you have no way of knowing if they are sterile. Do not use push-on type caps for hazardous materials. Twist-on caps are generally packaged singly, in packets similar to needles. The same technique used in applying a needle should be used to attach this type of cap to the syringe.

AUTOMATED COMPOUNDING DEVICES AND DISPENSING PUMPS

Several types of pumping systems are available to aid in compounding. There are some general considerations that apply to all compounders.

1. Compounders must be **cleaned, disinfected, and calibrated** prior to use.

2. **Tubing must be changed** at least as often as the manufacturer recommends. Be sure it is free of kinks and seated properly.

3. **Contamination of tubing at any time may result in contamination of every item compounded thereafter,** until the tubing is changed. Likewise, if an incorrect solution is attached, every item compounded will be wrong.

4. **Machines make errors.** The operator is responsible for verifying the proper operation of the compounder each and every time it dispenses.

5. If there is any doubt concerning the accuracy or purity of the compounded solution, it must be discarded.

6. Personnel must **complete training, testing, and validation** for each compounder they use, and manufacturer's instructions must be followed. All machines are slightly different. Do not assume you know how to use any unfamiliar equipment.

One-solution Pumps

The simplest devices pump one solution through one tube. These devices are usually calibrated volumetrically, and tend to drift with time because the tubing stretches, and should be recalibrated frequently. They should also be recalibrated when there is a significant change in the volume to be pumped because they are not calibrated over the entire span of possible volumes. They are not intended for use when precise measurements are required. These devices are best used for reconstituting single-dose vials, when the entire contents will be further diluted in a final bag, which will be fully administered. The following steps should be followed when using these devices:

1. When pumping from an unvented bottle, be sure the tubing vent is open.

2. Use a vented needle. Change the needle frequently and never use the same needle for reconstitution of different drugs.

3. Tests have shown that drug may aspirate into the tubing after pumping has finished. It is therefore recommended that the tubing be changed between reconstitution of different drugs. **If penicillin and other drugs frequently implicated in allergic reactions are reconstituted, the tubing must be changed.** The tubing should also be changed **if the diluent solution is changed.**

4. Recalibrate frequently.

Multiple-solution Compounders

Many pharmacies use automated compounders for Total Parenteral Nutrition (TPN) solutions, to which small volume components are then added. These compounders measure solutions gravimetrically, and have a higher degree of accuracy than the one-solution, volumetric pumps. However, several precautions must be taken when using an automated compounder for this purpose.

1. The tubing must be installed correctly. The supervising pharmacist must verify and document that the **color codes** for each station match the tubing.

2. The **correct solution** must be attached to each station. This must be verified by the supervising pharmacist, and should be checked on every shift and documented.

3. The **correct specific gravity** for each solution must be entered. The machine determines the weight of the solution to be pumped using the **volume entry** and the **specific gravity.** Both must be correct. Both must be verified by the pharmacist, and documented.

4. The compounder must be **calibrated** for both the **zero and span.** This must be documented and verified by the supervising pharmacist.

5. **Aseptic technique** must be used at all times when changing source containers, and when attaching the final solution bag. The cover of the connecting port must be closed when not in use. It is generally situated in a location which does not readily facilitate the flow of first air over this large, open orifice. Situate the compounder to maximize first air flow to this critical site.

6. The **correct spike adaptors** must be used for source solutions, particularly bottles.

7. The operator must **note the approximate volume in each source container** before and after pumping to verify that the correct volume was pumped.

Personnel often have the misconception that machines eliminate human error. This is not true. First, machines are set up and operated by humans, so, at best, you only substitute one type of human error for another. Second, the additional possibility of machine error is introduced. While automated compounders can be of great assistance in the pharmacy, the ultimate responsibility for **the quality of products compounded still rests with the individual operator, supported by the team.**

OTHER COMPOUNDING TOOLS

This manual describes techniques for many of the more commonly-encountered tools currently being used in pharmacy compounding. There are many that have not been discussed, and many new devices are currently in development. Always consult the manufacturer's instructions for use. However, manufacturers often cover aseptic manipulation of their instruments and devices with a statement that aseptic technique should be used, without elucidating how that is to be accomplished. The following steps are recommended for developing aseptic procedures for new and unfamiliar equipment and tools:

1. **Always** develop a written procedure. A team approach works best.

2. Consult the **manufacturer's instructions** and experiment with the device until you are certain you **understand how it works.**

3. **Define the task** for which the item will be used, and **identify all other items** which will be needed for the process.

4. Identify all **critical sites and pathways**.

5. Identify all **factors that effect accuracy.**

6. Identify all **hazards**.

7. Develop a step-by-step compounding procedure in a **flow chart, from staging to final check prior to release.**

8. On the flow chart, identify where the **critical sites and the operator's hands** are to be located at all times.

9. Have **each member of the team perform the initial draft procedure,** while the others observe. This will help identify manipulations which may be too difficult to be performed aseptically, accurately, or safely. Modify and trial the procedure until it is acceptable to everyone. Write down all observations and all changes that are developed so that you have a history of the process. **Define the engineering and barrier controls used to support the process.**

10. Identify the key aspects of the procedure, and **develop ways to monitor** for ongoing compliance with those aspects.

11. Formalize the procedure as a draft, and **train all operators** in the process.

12. **Perform a validation exercise.** The validation exercise should meet the following criteria:

    a. Products and batch sizes should be representative of the "worst-case" situation normally encountered (the most complex situation; largest number of repetitions).

b. It should be performed at the end of the shift, when operators are under the most stress, and most tired.

c. Sterile microbiologic growth media should be substituted for product, but extreme care must be taken and complete warning labeling must be used to keep the growth media out of the patient product stream. Complete line clearance, cleaning, and disinfection must be performed immediately following the exercise and documented.

d. Each operator should complete the exercise at least three times for minimum statistical reasons, and to demonstrate consistency.

e. The simulated microbiologic growth-media product should be given to the microbiology lab for incubation and observation.

13. If no growth occurs, adopt the procedure and monitoring plan. If growth occurs, an analysis must be made to identify the reason(s), and the procedure must be modified to eliminate the cause(s). The procedure must then be revalidated.

14. **Train and validate all new personnel, and revalidate all personnel and the process periodically,** including a written test of knowledge, derived from a written validation policy and procedure. Document all validation activities.

LABELING AND INITIALING

Upon completion of compounding, all labels should be applied and initialed by the operator. The date of compounding, as well as the solution expiration date should be noted. Any auxiliary labels, such as DO NOT REFRIGERATE, REFRIGERATE, and CHEMOTHERAPEUTIC AGENT warning labels should be attached. The final containers should be visually checked for particulates against both a white, and a black background. For hazardous materials, the bag should be wiped with a slightly moistened, low-lint wipe, and placed in a sealable plastic bag, appropriately labeled, prior to removal from the BSC. Identification and warning labels must be attached to the final product container, not just the outer bag, because this will eventually be removed.

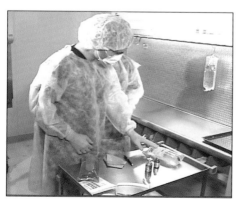

The final containers and vials should be presented to the pharmacist for the final check, and the pharmacist should also check for particulates. This redundancy will assure the best possible accuracy and surveillance of the product. When presenting hazardous materials vials for post-compounding cross-check, they should be sealed in a labeled plastic bag, oriented so the pharmacist can review all pertinent information.

POST-COMPOUNDING ACTIVITIES

All compounding debris and packaging materials should be disposed of properly. Be sure that ampules and syringes are placed in an appropriate sharps container, and residual fluids are carefully sealed in closed containers. All materials used in hazardous compounding procedures must be disposed of as contaminated waste in accordance with state and local regulations.

LINE CLEARANCE

Because many drugs may be a hazard to a patient for whom they are not intended, the line clearance is performed to assure that no drug or compounding residues remain in the critical work environment following the completion of compounding activities.

Any unused drugs, components, and labels should be removed from the compounding area. Unused components remaining in a BSC where hazardous materials have been compounded must be assumed to be contaminated, and cannot be returned to general storage areas. The hood work surfaces should be sanitized with a water-based, low-residuing disinfectant cleaner, followed by a 70% isopropanol or ethanol rinse, which is then allowed to dry. The undertray area of BSCs should be cleaned and disinfected. All line clearance activities should be documented.

Although this type of sanitizing is complete as a line clearance, it should be repeated again prior to the resumption of compounding activities if the operator leaves the compounding area for any reason, or when charge of the compounding area changes between shifts. It is not possible to know who, or what may have contaminated the critical work surfaces in your absence, and it cannot be assumed they have been properly sanitized by anyone else.

Self Evaluation: Aseptic Manipulations

1. The ideal percent of alcohol in water for disinfection of the critical worksurface is _____%. (Pages 30 and 34)

2. Regardless of how they appear, all Laminar flow devices should be sanitized prior to each use. (Page 33)

   True   False

3. In a horizontal LFCB, all working materials should be arranged front to back.(Page 40)

   True   False

4. A properly operating BSC will contain all hazardous contaminants and prevent contamination of the environment and personnel. (Page 41)

   True   False

5. Vacuum-packed glass bottles may be used, even if the vacuum is no longer intact, as long as the seals were intact when the container was opened. (Page 61)

   True   False

6. Emergency personnel are completely familiar with the chemotherapeutic agents used in hospitals. (Page 39)

   True   False

7. The document which describes the hazards of a drug, proper emergency treatment, and spill clean-up is called _____.(Page 39)

8. To keep paper-wrapped items, such as syringes and alcohol swabs out of the work zone of the BSC, you may lay them to one side of the hood on the front grill. (Page 41)

   True   False

9. First air is constantly flowing over the injection port of a bag hanging from the IV pole in a BSC. (Page 41)

   True   False

10. Gloves need to be disinfected each time the operator leaves the aseptic field. (Page 42)

    True   False

11. A water-based disinfectant should be used prior to alcohol disinfection because not all substances are _____ in alcohol. (Page 34)

12. Solutions in PVC plastic bags should be used within _____ _____ after removal of the outer bag, unless otherwise specified by the manufacturer. (Page 58)

13. It is acceptable to use the same syringe for several additives to one admixture, as long as syringe sterility is maintained. (Page 44)

True   False

14. Ampules should be broken toward the side of the hood to avoid damage to the _____. (Page 52)

15. Ampules may be reused if they are stored for a brief period of time directly in front of the HEPA filter. (Page 52)

True   False

16. To prevent coring, the needle should be _____ as it passes through the septum, so the bevel will be perpendicular to the septum. (Page 47)

17. Lower gauge needles are desirable in most situations because drug flows more freely and compounding is faster. (Page 42)

True   False

18. To get the last drops of drug from a vial, remove the dispensing pin and draw up the remainder with a syringe equipped with a filter needle. (Page 55)

True   False

19. Name three facts that must be verified based on the information on the label of an admixture component. _____, _____, and _____. (Page 39)

20. Handling the shaft of the syringe plunger is called _____ _____. (Page 43)

21. Alcohol is a disinfectant, not a sterilant. (Page 34)

True   False

22. Upon entry into the compounding area, verify that the hood cleaning logs were completed on the last shift, and that the hood is visibly clean. This eliminates the need for time-consuming recleaning. (Page 33)

True   False

23. The best way to remove fluids from a vial is to draw up air in the same volume as the required dose and inject it into the inverted vial so the drug will flow freely into the vial. (Page 48)

True   False

24. When compounding hazardous materials with a dispensing pin, the pin must have a _____ filter. (Page 44)

25. To assure accuracy when using an automated compounder, verify the _____ entry, the _____ entry, which determine the weight of solution pumped, and observe the pumping operation by checking the volume in the source container before and after pumping. (Page 64)

26. Describe the seven main steps for use of an ampule. (Pages 52 and 53)

     1) _____

     2) _____

     3) _____

     4) _____

     5) _____

     6) _____

     7) _____

27. Define plasmolysis and explain its application to aseptic compounding

_____

_____.

(Pages 31 and 34)

28. Wrap an ampule top with an alcohol swab to contain splatter and protect fingers. (Page 52)

                                                                  True   False

V. PHARMACEUTICAL CALCULATIONS

The pharmaceutical calculations presented incorporate standard algebraic expressions, and are intended as a general review of representative IV compounding exercises. Any student who experiences difficulty with these calculations should complete a basic orientation to pharmaceutical calculations using a competency-based text and workbook on pharmaceutical mathematics[15].

LEARNING OBJECTIVES FOR SECTION V.

Upon completion of this section you should:

Objective 5.1) Understand and solve problems using ratios, performing the basic mathematical functions on both the numeric, and unit of measure components of the equation.

Objective 5.2) Be able to convert from one unit of measure to another, and understand what is meant by significant digits.

Objective 5.3) Know the definition of percentage as it relates to pharmaceutical compounds and perform calculations using percentages.

Objective 5.4) Calculate administration and drip rates.

Objective 5.5) Perform dosage and dilution calculations.

Products may be admixed in the wrong amounts, effecting the efficacy and concentration of the drug(s). Therefore, performing certain types of mathematical calculations is integral to proper compounding of pharmaceutical products into finished dosage forms in pharmacy.

Even when computer systems perform calculations automatically, the pharmacist must still verify that all calculations were performed correctly, and the technician should cross-check all calculations to provide the highest possible assurance of accuracy. Computers do occasionally make errors, as their accuracy is dependent on data entered by humans.

RATIOS

Objective 5.1) Understand and solve problems using ratios, performing the basic mathematical functions on both the numeric, and unit of measure components of the expression.

Key Concept: Most calculations used in pharmacy can be expressed as ratios. Ratios are essentially fractions, and are manipulated according to the same rules. In a ratio, one quantity is related to another by a division operation.

Two ratios are equal to each other if dividing the numerator by the denominator results in the same value for both ratios.

$$\frac{2}{4} = \frac{5}{10} \quad \text{BECAUSE:}$$

Carrying out the divisions results in the value of 0.5 for both ratios.

PROBLEM SOLVING WITH RATIOS

To use ratios for problem solving, one ratio containing known information is set up as being equal to another ratio containing the unknown information. For example, to answer the question, "How many micrograms (mcg) are equal to 0.06 milligrams (mg)?", we set up the following equation, where the "how many" portion of the question is represented by the letter X (we can use any letter or non-numeric symbol to take the place of the unknown information in the equation).

STEP 1. SET UP AN EQUATION CONTAINING KNOWN AND UNKNOWN DATA

Using the known information and the fact that 1000 mcg are equal to 1 mg, we set up the following equation:

$$\frac{1000 \text{ mcg}}{1 \text{ mg}} = \frac{X \text{ mcg}}{0.06 \text{ mg}}$$

This statement can be read, "1000 mcg is **related to** 1 mg **as** X mcg **is related** to 0.06 mg.

STEP 2. ISOLATE THE UNKNOWN

The general approach to solving problems is to **isolate the unknown quantity on one side of the equation.** This should be done in a way that places the unknown in the numerator, not the denominator, which makes calculations much easier.

A general rule of calculations is that **both sides of an equation can be multiplied or divided by the same quantity without changing the value of the equation.**

Examining the equation above, we see that we can multiply both sides by 0.06 mg, which will leave X mcg alone on one side of the equation in the numerator.

$$(0.06 \text{ mg}) \quad \frac{1000 \text{ mcg}}{1 \text{ mg}} \quad = \quad \frac{X \text{ mcg}}{0.06 \text{ mg}} \quad (0.06 \text{ mg})$$

STEP 3. SIMPLIFY THE EQUATION

Any quantity **divided by itself** is equal to **one.** Because a quantity in the numerator is being divided by a quantity in the denominator, multiplication factors found in both the numerator and denominator can be "cancelled". (NOTE: Quantities to be **added to** or **subtracted from** other quantities *cannot* be cancelled.) Cancel the **mg** on both sides, and the **0.06** in the right side of the equation. Let the ones in the denominators be understood. We can do this because division of any quantity by one results in the quantity, itself. After this is accomplished, simple mathematical operations will provide the solution.

$$(0.06 \text{ mg}) \quad \frac{1000 \text{ mcg}}{1 \text{ mg}} \quad = \quad \frac{X \text{ mcg}}{\textbf{0.06 mg}} \quad (\textbf{0.06 mg})$$

STEP 4. PERFORM CALCULATIONS

$$(0.06)(1000 \text{ mcg}) = X \text{ mcg}$$

Multiply the 0.06 by 1000.

$$60 \text{ mcg} = X \text{ mcg}$$

The answer is 60 mcg = X mcg.

Notice that the units of measure are manipulated in exactly **the same way as the numbers in an equation.** Always carry out the unit of measure calculations. It is an excellent way to verify that the manipulations were performed properly. If the units don't come out the way they should, the answer is probably wrong.

SAMPLE PROBLEM

A patient weighing 76.2 kilograms (kg) is to receive 0.24 units (u) of insulin per kg of weight in a solution which will be administered over the course of 24 hours. How many units of insulin are required for the solution?

What is known?	a) The patient is to receive 0.24 u per kg over 24 hours.
	b) The patient weighs 76.2 kg.
What is unknown?	**The total number of units the patient is to receive.**

STEP 1. SET UP THE EQUATION

Let X u = the total number of units, and set up two equivalent ratios. The known ratio is expressed as "0.24 u per kg". The unknown number of units has the same relationship to the total weight (76.2 kg) as 0.24 u has to 1 kg.

$$\frac{0.24 \text{ u}}{1 \text{ kg}} = \frac{X \text{ u}}{76.2 \text{ kg}}$$

STEP 2. ISOLATE THE UNKNOWN

Multiply both sides of the equation by 76.2 kg.

$$(76.2 \text{ kg}) \; \frac{0.24 \text{ u}}{1 \text{ kg}} = \frac{X \text{ u}}{76.2 \text{ kg}} \; (76.2 \text{ kg})$$

STEP 3. SIMPLIFY THE EXPRESSION

Cancel the **kg** on both sides of the equation, and the **76.2** on the right side. Let the ones in the denominator be understood.

$$(76.2 \; \textbf{kg}) \; \frac{0.24 \text{ u}}{1 \; \textbf{kg}} = \frac{X \text{ u}}{76.2 \; \textbf{kg}} \; (76.2 \; \textbf{kg})$$

STEP 4. PERFORM CALCULATIONS

Perform the multiplication of 76.2 X 0.24 u on the left side of the equation. The resulting answer is 18.3 units.

CONVERSION OF UNITS OF MEASURE

Objective 5.2) Be able to convert from one unit of measure to another, and understand what is meant by significant digits.

Key Concept: A conversion factor is a special kind of ratio that is equal to one, and is used to convert units of measure. An example is, "There are 1000 micrograms (mcg) per milligram (mg)", which is written:

$$\frac{1000 \text{ mcg}}{1 \text{ mg}}$$

It can also be written one milligram per one thousand micrograms.

$$\frac{1000 \text{ mcg}}{1\text{mg}} \qquad \frac{1 \text{ mg}}{1000 \text{ mcg}}$$

In either case, the expression is equal to 1, and can be inserted as a multiplier into any calculation, in either order, without changing the value of the calculation.

$$\frac{1000 \text{ mcg}}{1\text{mg}} = 1 \qquad \frac{1 \text{ mg}}{1000 \text{ mcg}} = 1$$

Use conversion factors that will allow unwanted units of measure to cancel, leaving only the units of measure that are appropriate to the desired answer. In other words, if the answer should be expressed in mcg, and the expression containing mg is in the numerator, use the first expression, placing the unwanted mg in the denominator to make cancellation possible. If the unwanted mg is in the denominator, choose the second version, placing the mg in the numerator to permit cancellation.

To convert from one unit of measure to another, obtain a "conversion ratio" from a chart, set up an equation using known and unknown data, and solve for the unknown.

SAMPLE PROBLEM

A medicine cup contains 2-1/2 ounces of liquid having a Sp.Gv. of 1.0, and you want to know how many grams it contains. Convert 2-1/2 ounces (oz) to grams (g).

Change the 1/2 to a decimal by dividing 1 by 2. Thus, 2-1/2 becomes 2.5. Next, go to a chart and find that there are 28.35 grams per ounce. Let X grams represent the unknown.

STEP 1. SET UP THE EQUATION

Set up an equation for X grams using the known information. "28.35 grams *is related to* 1 ounce *as* X grams *is related to* 2.5 ounces."

$$\frac{28.35 \text{ g}}{1 \text{ oz}} = \frac{X \text{ g}}{2.5 \text{ oz}}$$

STEP 2. ISOLATE THE UNKNOWN

Multiply both sides of the equation by 2.5 ounces to isolate the unknown.

$$(\textbf{2.5 oz}) \ \frac{28.35 \text{ g}}{1 \text{ oz}} = \frac{X \text{ g}}{\textbf{2.5 oz}} \ (\textbf{2.5 oz})$$

STEP 3. SIMPLIFY THE EXPRESSION

Cancel the **oz** on both sides of the equation and the **2.5** on the right side.

STEP 4. PERFORM CALCULATIONS

Perform the calculation, and let the ones be understood. The solution calculated is 70.875g = X grams. However, this answer is not acceptable in the form written. It violates the "**rule of significant digits**", which states that **no answer can express a higher degree of accuracy than the least accurate term used in the calculation.** The degree of accuracy can be generally interpreted as the number of decimal places. There is only 1 decimal place in 2.5 oz, therefore, there can be only one decimal place in the final answer. Look at the digit immediately to the right of the last acceptable significant decimal place (in this case, the one-hundredths place). Because the number in the one-hundredths place is greater than five, we round up to 70.9g. If it were less than five, we would round down.

SAMPLE PROBLEM

A patient weighs 176 pounds, but the dosage is given in micrograms per kilogram of weight. What is the patient's weight in kilograms?

STEP 1. SET UP THE EQUATION

Look in a table and find the conversion factor "1 kilogram equals 2.2 pounds".

$$\frac{X \text{ kg}}{176 \text{ Lb}} = \frac{1 \text{ kg}}{2.2 \text{ Lb}}$$

STEP 2. ISOLATE THE UNKNOWN

Multiply both sides of the equation by **2.2 Lb** and **176** to eliminate the fractional expressions and isolate the unknown.

$$(\textbf{2.2 Lb})(\textbf{176}) \quad \frac{X \text{ kg}}{\textbf{176 Lb}} = \frac{1 \text{ kg}}{\textbf{2.2 Lb}} \quad (\textbf{2.2 Lb})(\textbf{176})$$

STEPS 3 and 4. SIMPLIFY THE EXPRESSION AND PERFORM CALCULATIONS

Cancel the **Lb** on both sides, the **176** on the left side, and the **2.2** on the right side. Let the ones in the denominator be understood.

$$(2.2) \, X \text{ kg} = 1 \text{ kg} \, (176)$$

Divide by 2.2 to isolate the unknown. The answer is 80 kg.

PERCENTAGE CALCULATIONS

Objective 5.3) Know the definition of percentage as it relates to pharmaceutical compounds and perform calculations using percentages.

Key Concept: Percentages are a special kind of ratio (decimal fraction) with a denominator of 100, which are represented in mathematical shorthand as %. The word percent means "per 100". In other words, 5% is actually 5/100, or 0.05. This means that, if a whole object is divided into 100 parts, the fraction or decimal represents five of those parts. We are interested in working with percentages because the concentration of drug in many pharmaceutical preparations is expressed as a percentage. Unlike more commonly-encountered percentages, pharmaceutical percentage expressions have special meanings based on the form the drug is provided in. In particular, percentages involving the amount of a solid suspended or dissolved in a liquid must be properly interpreted to calculate the correct quantity required in an admixture.

CONVERSION OF DECIMALS TO PERCENTAGES

To convert a decimal to a percentage, multiply by 100 and add a percent sign.

CONVERSION OF FRACTIONS TO PERCENTAGES

To convert a fraction to a percentage you must first convert it to a decimal fraction by dividing the denominator into the numerator.

SAMPLE PROBLEM

Convert **1/16** to a percentage.

Dividing **1** by **16** results in the decimal fraction **0.0625**.

Multiplication by **100** and addition of the percent sign yields the value 6.25%.

Notice that a percentage can have decimal places in it. Also, **moving the decimal point** two **places to the** right is the same as multiplying by **100**. Conversely, **moving the decimal point two places to the left** is the same as **dividing** by **100.**

You may by wondering what happened to the rule of significant digits in this example because there were no decimal places in the expression 1/16 but there are four in the decimal fraction, and two in the percentage expression.

Key Concept: The rule of significant digits applies to calculations involving measurements, which can be no more precise than the least precise measurement used in the calculation. It is intended to prevent over-confidence in the precision of a number, while preserving the precision required and provided by the measurements. **This example is a purely numeric calculation of the value of a fraction, expressed as a decimal.**

The rule of significant digits should be adhered to in pharmaceutical calculations because the degree of precision in the dosage ordered may be required to properly treat the patient. If an order called for 0.08mg/kg/min, rounding up to 0.1 mg would result in **a 25% overdose.**

Conversely, in the example where 2.5 ounces was converted to grams, the least significant digit was in the ounces expression, and reflects the degree of accuracy of a measurement. Extreme care must also be exercised when placing the "**deadly** decimal point". It is very easy to misplace the decimal point by one place, which results in a **10-fold error.** Calculations should be carefully cross-checked for this reason, if no other.

PHARMACEUTICAL PERCENTAGE EXPRESSIONS

There are three basic types of percentage expressions used to define the concentration of pharmaceutical preparations, including weight-to-weight (W/W), weight-to-volume (W/V), and volume-to-volume (V/V) relationships.

Weight-to-Weight Percentage Expressions

Because solids are more easily weighed than measured volumetrically, for mixtures of solids, percentage means parts by weight of a drug in parts by weight of the mixture. (Percent weight-to-weight, **W/W**, equals the number of **grams** of the substance **per 100 grams** of mixture.)

$$\text{Percent weight-to-weight (W/W)} = \frac{\text{Number of grams of substance}}{100 \text{ grams of mixture}}$$

Weight-to-Volume Percentage Expressions

Because liquids are more easily measured volumetrically than weighed, for mixtures of solids in liquids, percentage means parts by weight of a drug in parts by volume of mixture. (Percent weight-to-volume, **W/V**, equals the number of **grams** of the substance **per 100 milliliters** of mixture.)

$$\text{Percent weight-to-volume (W/V)} = \frac{\text{number of grams of substance}}{100 \text{ milliliters of mixture}}$$

Volume-to-Volume Percentage Expressions

For mixtures of liquids in liquids, percentage means parts by volume of a drug in parts by volume of the mixture. (Percent volume-to-volume, **V/V**, equals the number of **milliliters** of the substance **per 100 milliliters** of mixture.)

$$\text{Percent volume-to-volume (V/V)} = \frac{\text{number of mL of substance}}{100 \text{ milliliters of mixture}}$$

Basic Rules For Solving Percentage Problems:

Rule 1: To perform calculations with percentages, you must first **convert them to decimals**. Remember, to convert a percentage to a decimal, **divide by 100** (move the decimal point **two places to the left**) and remove the % sign.

Rule 2: The quantities of the active ingredient and the total amounts must always be in the required units of measure. **Use grams for solids** and **milliliters for liquids.** Use standard conversion factors to convert to grams and milliliters.

The fundamental percentage equation can be written as follows, with calculations performed to convert to, or from a percentage as defined above:

$$\text{Percentage Strength} = \frac{\text{Amount of Active Ingredient}}{\text{Total Weight or Volume of Mixture}}$$

SAMPLE PROBLEM

Find the amount of the active ingredient when the percentage strength and the total quantity of the mixture are known.

How many grams of zinc oxide are there in 120 g of 20% zinc oxide ointment? Let X represent the "How many" part of the question.

STEP 1. SET UP THE EQUATION

In this case, we only need to make substitutions into the standard equation.

$$\text{(Percentage Strength) } 20\% = \frac{\text{X g (Amount of Active Ingredient)}}{\text{120 g (Total Weight or Volume of Mixture)}}$$

STEP 2. ISOLATE THE UNKNOWN

Multiply by 120 g to isolate the unknown and eliminate the fractional expression.

$$(120 \text{ g}) (20\%) = \text{X g}$$

STEP 3. SIMPLIFY

Convert the percentage side of the expression by dividing by 100 and removing the percent sign.

$$(120 \text{ g}) (0.20) = X \text{ g}$$

STEP 4. PERFORM CALCULATIONS

Carry out the calculation by multiplying 120 g by 0.20.

$$X \text{ g} = 24 \text{ g}$$

Similar substitutions can be made to find the total quantity of a mixture when the percentage strength and the amount of the active ingredient are known, or the percentage strength when the amount of active ingredient and total volume are known.

These calculations are simple, however, it is very easy to forget to convert to grams and milliliters, or to inadvertently perform the calculation based on parts of substance per liter or kilogram, rather than per 100 mL or 100 g. Exercise extreme care when performing these calculations because it is one of the easiest ways to misplace the "**deadly decimal point**".

SAMPLE PROBLEM

A 70% alcohol/water solution contains 55 mL of pure alcohol. What is the total volume of the solution?

STEP 1. SET UP EQUATION BY SUBSTITUTION

$$70\% = \frac{55 \text{ mL}}{X \text{ mL}}$$

STEP 2. ISOLATE THE UNKNOWN

Multiply by **X mL** to eliminate the fractional expression, and divide by **70%** to isolate the unknown.

$$\frac{(X \text{ mL}) (\textbf{70\%})}{\textbf{70\%}} = \frac{(55 \text{ mL}) (\textbf{X mL})}{(\textbf{X mL}) (70\%)}$$

STEP 3. SIMPLIFY

Divide by 100 and remove the % sign to convert to a decimal.

$$X \text{ mL} = \frac{55 \text{ mL}}{0.70}$$

STEP 4. PERFORM CALCULATIONS

The result of the calculation is X = 78.57. However, this expression is not the correct answer. There are no decimal places in 55 mL, so there cannot be any decimal places in the answer. The last significant digit is the "ones" place. The numeral to the right of the last significant digit is 5. When this occurs we can round up or down. One convention is to round which ever way produces an even number, so in this case we will round down to 78 mL.

SAMPLE PROBLEM

Find the percentage strength of a solution containing 246 g of Dextrose in 1 liter (L) of Sterile Water for Injection U.S.P.

STEP 1. SET UP THE EQUATION BY SUBSTITUTION

$$X\% = \frac{246 \text{ g}}{1 \text{ L}}$$

Remember that rule two says to express all quantities in grams and milliliters. The expression becomes:

$$X\% = \frac{246 \text{ g}}{1000 \text{ mL}}$$

STEP 2. ISOLATE THE UNKNOWN

In this equation, the unknown is already isolated.

STEP 3. SIMPLIFY

Because the final answer is to be expressed as a percentage, no simplification is required.

STEP 4. PERFORM THE CALCULATIONS

Calculation of the right side of the equation yields the answer 0.246 g/mL. A decimal is converted to a percentage by multiplying by one hundred and adding a percent sign which results in:

$$X\% = 24.6\%.$$

Because these calculations simply convert the degree of accuracy represented by the measurement of 246 g in 1 liter to another method of notation, the rule of significant digits does not apply. Rounding up to 25% would lead to an erroneously inexact answer. **Remember, the objective of the rule of significant digits is to assure that the mathematical expression reflects the actual degree of accuracy of the measurements.**

ADMINISTRATION AND DRIP RATES

Objective 5.4) Calculate administration and drip rates.

Administration and drip rates are easily calculated using ratio equations, because a rate is a ratio expressing volume to be administered **per** time. Administration rate is determined by the following equation:

$$\text{Administration Rate} = \frac{\text{Total Volume to be infused}}{\text{Infusion Time}}$$

SAMPLE PROBLEM

Find the total length of time an IV solution containing 1000 mL will run if the flow rate is 70 mL per hour.

STEP 1. SET UP THE EQUATION BY SUBSTITUTION

$$\frac{70 \text{ mL}}{1 \text{ hour}} = \frac{1000 \text{ mL}}{X \text{ hour}}$$

First multiply by X hr to place the unknown in the numerator.

STEPS 2, 3, AND 4. ISOLATE THE UNKNOWN, SIMPLIFY, and PERFORM CALCULATIONS

$$(X \text{ hr}) \quad \frac{(70 \text{ mL})}{\text{hr}} \quad = 1000 \text{ mL}$$

Cancel the **hr** on the left side, then divide by 70mL to isolate the unknown: X = 14.3, which becomes 14 when the rule of significant digits is applied.

CONVERSION TO DROPS PER MINUTE

To find the flow rate as drops per minute instead of mL per hour, convert mL/hr to mL/min by dividing 70 milliliters per hour by 60 minutes per hour, which equals X milliliters per minute.

$$\frac{70 \text{ mL/hour}}{60 \text{ min/hour}} \quad = \quad X \text{ mL/min}$$

To simplify the calculations you may separate multiplication factors. The expression becomes 70 ***times*** **milliliters per hour**, divided by 60 ***times*** **minutes per hour.**

$$\frac{(70) \, (\text{mL/hr})}{(60) \, (\text{min/hr})} \quad = \quad X \text{ mL/min}$$

The expression can be further rewritten as follows:

$$\frac{70 \bullet \dfrac{\text{mL}}{\text{hr}}}{60 \bullet \dfrac{\text{min}}{\text{hr}}} \quad = X \text{ mL/min}$$

When the denominator is a fraction as **minutes per hour** is in this example, the rule is to **invert the denominator, and multiply**. The expression then becomes:

$$\frac{70}{60} \quad \bullet \quad \frac{\text{mL}}{\text{hr}} \quad \bullet \quad \frac{\text{hr}}{\text{min}} \quad = \quad X \text{ mL/min}$$

The **hours** cancel, and 70 divided by 60 equals 1.17, therefore the administration rate expressed in mL/min is 1.17. We need to know this because the drip rate is expressed in drops per mL, and we want to know how many drops per minute are required to achieve the desired administration rate. Each administration set has a conversion factor for its drip chamber written on its container. The following are common drip rates:

Standard administration set: 10 drops = 1 mL

Minidrip administration set: 60 drops = 1 mL

Convert mL/minute to drops/minute in the last equation for a standard set with a drip rate of 10 drops per mL.

$$1.17 \ \frac{\mathbf{mL}}{\min} \bullet 10 \ \frac{\text{drops}}{\mathbf{mL}} = X \ \frac{\text{drops}}{\min}$$

The mL cancel. Carry out the calculation. The answer is 11.7 drops per minute, which becomes 12 when the rule of significant digits is applied. Notice that we did not round off 1.17 mL/min. When performing a series of calculations, let the non-significant decimal places run until the final calculation so that you are not rounding off numbers based on calculations made with rounded off numbers.

Many personnel are quite capable of performing calculations in their head, without writing down all of the intermediate steps we have defined. There are several reasons you should get in the habit of writing out all calculations, including units of measure and intermediate steps. First, this practice makes it much easier to check calculations. Second, as was mentioned, including the units of measure assists in the recognition of errors. The most important reason, however, is to make **absolutely sure** that the **deadly decimal point** is in the correct location.

DOSAGE AND DILUTION CALCULATIONS

Objective 5.5) Perform dosage and dilution calculations.

Key Concept: Dosage and dilution calculations determine the amount of drug a patient receives, and **must** be accurate.

Dosage and dilution calculations are solved by setting up one or more equations using ratios. It is useful to remember that all "conversion ratios" are, by definition, equal to one, and can be inserted as multipliers anywhere to change units, in either order.

SAMPLE PROBLEM

A Total Parenteral Nutrition (TPN) solution is to deliver 8 milliequivalents (mEq) of Magnesium sulfate per liter, which is supplied as a 50% solution. How many mL of solution are required for a 2 liter TPN.

Start with an equation using the known information and let X equal the mL of solution required. A 50% solution contains 50 grams per 100 mL of solution.

$$\frac{8 \text{ mEq}}{1 \text{ L}} \bullet \frac{50 \text{ g}}{100 \text{ mL}} \bullet \frac{1000 \text{ mg}}{1 \text{ g}} \bullet 2 \text{ L} = X \text{ mL}$$

Cancel L, g, and 100, and carry out the calculations.

$$\frac{8 \text{ mEq}}{1 \textbf{ L}} \bullet \frac{50 \textbf{ g}}{100 \text{ mL}} \bullet \frac{1000 \text{ mg}}{1 \textbf{g}} \bullet 2 \textbf{ L} = X \text{ mL}$$

$$\frac{8 \bullet \textbf{ mEq} \bullet 50 \bullet 10 \bullet \textbf{ mg} \bullet 2}{\text{mL}} = X \text{ mL}$$

$$\frac{8 \bullet 2 \bullet 50 \bullet 10 \bullet \textbf{ mEq} \bullet \textbf{ mg}}{\text{mL}} = X \text{ mL}$$

We have hit a dead end. By carrying out operations on the units of measure, we are able to see clearly that we have done something wrong. In order to solve the equation as set up, you would need a conversion factor for mEq and mg. However, the equivalent weight of a substance is based upon the molecular weight of the substance and the valance of the atom(s), (some elements may have more than one valance) and must be calculated from the atomic chart based upon a complete understanding of the molecule's configuration. **The weight (mass) and volume of one equivalent or one mole is different for every substance.** The term "normal" is based upon the equivalent weight of the substance, also. Therefore, a normal of one substance is not equal in weight to a normal of another. Remember: **No single conversion factor exists for converting equivalent weights, molar concentrations or normals to conventional measures of weight.** To solve this problem, we need to know that each mL of the MgSO$_4$ contains 4.06mEq. The problem is then solved as follows:

$$X \text{ mL} = \frac{8 \text{ mEq}}{1 \text{ L}} \bullet 2 \text{ L} \bullet \frac{1 \text{ mL}}{4.06 \text{ mEq}}$$

Cancel the liters and milliequivalents and perform the calculation. The solution requires 3.94 mL of MgSO$_4$, which becomes 4 mL when the rule of significant digits is applied.

SAMPLE PROBLEM

The most complex solutions normally encountered in pharmacy compounding are Total Parenteral Nutrition (TPN) solutions. The pharmacist and physician determine the composition of the TPN, but accuracy is essential, and the calculations should be verified. *All of the skills you have developed are required for these calculations.*

The final volume of a TPN is 1800 mL, and will run for 12 hours using an administration set with a 10 drops per minute drip rate. The patient weight is 24.6 kg.

Component solutions include:

Amino Acid Solution	10%
Dextrose	70%
Intralipid	20%
Sodium Chloride	100 mEq/40.0 mL
Potassium Phosphates	
Potassium	3 mM/mL
Phosphates	4.4 mEq/mL
Magnesium Sulfate	50%, 4.06 mEq/mL
Heparin	1000 u/mL
Calcium Gluconate	10%, 0.465 mEq Ca/mL

as well as MVI 9+3, Pedtrace, and sterile water for injection. Calculate the volumes of each component required to achieve the following concentrations:

Component	Ordered
Amino Acid Solution	2 gm/kg
Dextrose	17.5%
Intralipid	2.25 gm/kg
Sodium Chloride	26 mEq/liter

Potassium Phosphates	26 mEq/liter phosphates
Magnesium Sulfate	8 mEq/liter
Heparin	1000 u/liter
Calcium Gluconate	1000 mg
MVI 9+3	5 mL
Pedtrace	0.2 mL/kg
Sterile Water	QS to 1800 mL

Amino Acid Solution   2 g/kg

For each calculation, begin with the **quantity ordered. Multiply** by the quantity which determines the amount required, usually either the **patient weight** or the **total volume of the final solution. Multiply** by the concentration of the source solution.

(Ordered)(times)(patient weight)(times)(source % in mL and grams)

$$2\,\frac{g}{kg} \quad \bullet \quad 24.6\ \text{kg} \quad \bullet \quad \frac{100\ \text{mL}}{10\ \text{g}} = 492\ \text{mL}$$

Note that we inverted the concentration of Amino Acid Solution. Ten percent (W/V) means 10 g per 100 mL, but it also means 100 mL per 10 g. Writing it this way makes the calculation easier because the grams cancel and the answer is in mL as needed. Writing out calculations makes it easier to identify the order in which expressions should be written and also makes it easier for others to cross-check your work.

Dextrose   17.5%

(Ordered per 1000 mL)(times)(total volume)(times)(source % in g and mL)

$$\frac{175\ \text{g}}{1000\ \text{mL}} \quad \bullet \quad 1800\ \text{mL} \quad \bullet \quad \frac{100\ \text{mL}}{70\ \text{g}} = 450\ \text{mL}$$

Intralipid   2.25 g/kg

(Ordered g/weight)(times)(weight)(times)(source % in milliliters and grams)

$$2.25\,\frac{g}{kg} \quad \bullet \quad 24.6\ \text{kg} \quad \bullet \quad \frac{100\ \text{mL}}{20\ \text{g}} = 277\ \text{mL}$$

Sodium Chloride   26 mEq/liter

(Amount ordered/1000 mL)(times)(total volume)(times)(source concentration)

$$\frac{26\ \textbf{mEq}}{1000\ \textbf{mL}} \quad \bullet \quad 1800\ \text{mL} \quad \bullet \quad \frac{40\ \text{mL}}{100\ \textbf{mEq}} = 19\ \text{mL}$$

Potassium Phosphates   26 mEq/liter phosphate

(Amount ordered/1000 mL)(times)(total volume)(times)(source concentration)

$$\frac{26\ \textbf{mEq}}{1000\ \textbf{mL}} \quad \bullet \quad 1800\ \text{mL} \quad \bullet \quad \frac{1\ \text{mL}}{4.4\ \textbf{mEq}} = 11\ \text{mL}$$

Magnesium Sulfate   8 mEq/liter

(Amount ordered/1000 mL)(times)(total volume)(times)(source concentration)

$$\frac{8\ \textbf{mEq}}{1000\ \textbf{mL}} \quad \bullet \quad 1800\ \text{mL} \quad \bullet \quad \frac{\text{mL}}{4.06\ \textbf{mEq}} = 4\ \text{mL}$$

Heparin   1000 u/liter

(Amount ordered/1000 mL)(times)(total volume)(times)(source concentration)

$$\frac{1000\ \text{u}}{1000\ \textbf{mL}} \quad \bullet \quad 1800\ \text{mL} \quad \bullet \quad \frac{1\ \text{mL}}{1000\ \text{u}} = 1.8\ \text{mL}$$

Calcium Gluconate   1000 mg

(Ordered)(times)(Convert ordered to g from mg)(times)(convert % to g and mL)

$$1000\ \textbf{mg} \quad \bullet \quad \frac{1\ \text{g}}{1000\ \textbf{mg}} \quad \bullet \quad \frac{100\ \text{mL}}{10\ \text{g}} = 10\ \text{mL}$$

MVI 9+3   **5 mL**

Pedtrace   **0.2 mL/kg**

(Ordered per weight)(times)(patient weight)

$$0.2 \ \frac{mL}{kg} \quad \bullet \quad 24.6 \ \textbf{kg} \ = 4.9 \ mL$$

Sterile Water   **QS to 1800 mL**

Total volume of all other components is 1275 mL, therefore, 525 mL of water are required to achieve the final solution volume of 1800 mL. The total solution volume is divided by 12 to determine the mL/hr administration rate(150), and this is divided by 60 to determine mL/min (2.5). Multiply by 10 drops per mL to determine the drip rate per minute, which is 25 drops per minute.

Self Evaluation: Pharmaceutical Calculations

1. If the drip rate of an administration set is 60 drops per mL and a 336 mL solution is to run for 24 hours, what is the required drip rate per minute? _____.

2. A 1 liter solution is to contain 0.2 g of Magnesium Sulfate, and 3.5 mEq of Potassium Chloride. Component solution concentrations are as follows:

Magnesium Sulfate   50%   4.06 mEq/mL
Potassium Chloride   60 mEq/30mL

Calculate the volumes required of each component listed above:

Component   Ordered   Required Volume

Magnesium Sulfate   0.2 g/liter
Potassium Chloride   3.5 mEq/liter

3. (10 points) Express the following as milligrams:

a) 1 g = _____ b) 0.25 g= _____ c) 2 g= _____ d) 2/3 g = _____

e) 1/2 g = _____ f) 22 mcg = _____ g) 725 mcg= _____

4. (10 points) Express the following as percentages:

a) 180 g in 250 mL = _____ b) 27 g in 1 liter = _____

c) 1/8 = _____ d) 1.634 = _____ e) 1/12 = _____

f) 25 g in 2 kg = _____ g) 23 mL in 2 liters = _____

5. A patient weighing 4.5 kg is to receive a 336 mL TPN. It is to be compounded from the following components:

Amino Acid Solution	10%
Dextrose	70%
Intralipid	20%
Sodium Chloride	100 mEq/40mL
Potassium Chloride	2 mEq/mL
Potassium Phosphates	
Potassium	3 mM/mL
Phosphates	4.4 mEq/mL
Magnesium Sulfate	50%, 4.06 mEq/mL
Heparin	1000 u/mL
Calcium Gluconate	10%, 0.465 mEq Ca/mL

Calculate the volumes required of each component to achieve the following:

Component	Ordered	Required Volume
Amino Acid Solution	2.5 gm/kg	
Dextrose	17.5%	
Intralipid	2.13 gm/kg	
Sodium Chloride	35 mEq/liter	
Potassium Chloride	20 mEq/liter	
Potassium Phosphates	26 mEq/liter phosphate	
Magnesium Sulfate	8 mEq/liter	
Heparin	1000 u/liter	
Calcium Gluconate	100 mg/kg	
Sterile Water	QS to 1800 mL	

ANSWERS TO SELF-EVALUATIONS

Part I: Quality Assurance Theory for IV Admixtures

1. touch
2. false
3. pathogens
4. pyrogens
5. product is contaminated drug residues.
6. acceptable quality limits
7. aseptic processing
8. skin; gut; lungs; vascularized epithelia
9. parenteral
10. potential
11. transfer
12. events
13. individual, team

Part II: Engineering Controls and Laminar Airflow Theory

1. first air
2. speed, direction
3. airborne
4. backwash
5. downstream
6. cross-stream
7. smoke-split
8. b
9. false
10. 90
11. primary, secondary
12. false
13. aluminum separators
14. primary
15. 99.97%
16. zone, confusion
17. false
18. cleaner; dirtier
19. false
20. false

Part III: Barrier Controls

1. false
2. false
3. false
4. true
5. gloves; mask; gown; hair cover; shoe covers; goggles
6. true
7. false
8. false

Part IV: Aseptic Manipulations

1. 70%
2. true
3. false
4. false
5. false
6. false
7. Material Safety Data Sheet
8. false
9. false
10. true

11. soluble
12. 30 days
13. false
14. HEPA filter
15. false
16. bowed
17. false
18. false
19. Identity; concentration; expiry date
20. palming the plunger
21. true
22. false
23. false

24. hydrophobic
25. specific gravity; volume
26. check label, container & contents
    remove drug from neck
    clean and disinfect neck
    assemble syringe
    snap open facing side of hood
    draw up contents
    filter contents
27. cell membrane destruction caused by
    alcohol drying required for effective
    disinfection
28. false

Part V: Compounding Calculations
1. 14

2. $MgSO_4$ = 0.4 mL; KCl = 2 mL

3. a. 1000
    b. 250
    c. 2000
    d. 667
    e. 500
    f. 0.022
    g. 0.725

4. a. 72%
    b. 2.7%
    c. 12.5%
    d. 163.4%
    e. 8.3%
    f. 1.25%
    g. 1.15%

5. 112 mL, 84 mL, 48 mL, 5 mL, 3 mL, 2 mL, 1 mL, 0.3 mL, 4 mL,
    77 mL

CRITERIA FOR PRACTICAL EVALUATION

1. The Standard for acceptable performance is 90% compliance with technique.

2. The practical evaluation consists of manipulation of Sterile Microbiologic Growth Media. Microbiologic contamination of any of the products prepared automatically results in failure. Additionally, performance is observed for the following:

3. Proper pre-cleaning and sanitizing of the hoods.

4. Proper hygiene and gowning.

5. Proper staging of materials in the hood.

6. Manipulations performed using good aseptic technique including, but are not limited to:

      a. Proper disinfection of critical sites
      b. Maintenance of first air to all critical sites.
      c. Aseptic handling of all compounding materials
      d. Proper selection and handling of syringes and needles.
      e. Proper disinfection of ampule
      f. Correct technique when opening ampule
      g. All preparations made prior to opening ampule
      h. Ampule contents filtered.
      i. No excessive or abrupt movements
      j. Proper handling of waste and product
      k. No practices that lead to coring or large needle holes.

THE AUTHORS

MARGHI R. McKEON is the Director of Quality Assurance for Lab Safety Corporation, and has been responsible for educational program development and administration since 1989. Ms. McKeon received her undergraduate degree in Biology and Chemistry from the University of Wisconsin, Eau Claire, in 1983. She has pursued additional graduate studies in biology and education, concentrating on programs for adult learners.

Prior to assuming her current position, Ms. McKeon served as the Quality Assurance Manager for a pharmaceutical manufacturer, was manager of an electron microscopy laboratory for a major metropolitan medical center, and conducted grant-funded basic research for the food-processing industry. Ms. McKeon authored "Ultrastructure of the Scutellum in Zea mays" (Wisc. Acad. of Arts, Sciences, and Letters, 1983), "Behavior of Euphorbia sativa in Liquid Tissue Culture" (proprietary, 1984), and co-authored "Microbiologic Monitoring of Aseptic and Controlled Processes", Vol. 19, The Encyclopedia of Pharmaceutical Technology (2000). She is currently preparing an additional article to appear in the online EPT Second Edition and desk-reference in the year 2001.

GREGORY F. PETERS founded the Lab Safety Corporation in 1979 as a firm specializing in contamination-control design and validation, and is responsible for all process and facility design and validation for radioneuclides, radiopharmaceuticals, antineoplastics, biohazards, and Pharmacy-dispensed sterile products. Mr. Peters completed the Hospital Medication Technician Certification Program at Rush University in 1965, and assumed responsibility for administration of all medications to patients on a Hematology/Oncology floor at the Rush-Presbyterian-St. Luke's Medical Center, Chicago. He received his undergraduate degree in Aviation Technology from Central Texas College in 1970.

Mr. Peters has written numerous works, including: "A Validation and Monitoring System for Pharmacy-produced IV Admixtures" (proprietary; 1980), "Laminar Airflow Equipment: Engineering Control of Aseptic Processing", Vol. 8, The Encyclopedia of Pharmaceutical Technology (1993), and co-authored "Microbiologic Monitoring of Aseptic and Controlled Processes", The Encyclopedia of Pharmaceutical Technology (2000). He is currently preparing additional articles to appear in the online EPT Second Edition and desk-reference in the year 2001.

REFERENCES

1. *Code of Federal Regulations,* Title 21, Part 211, *The Good Manufacturing Practices.* U.S. Government Printing Office, Washington D.C.

2. Turco, S. J., "Sterile Dosage Forms: their preparation and clinical application." 4th Ed., Lea and Febiger, Philadelphia. 1993.

3. Center for Drugs and Biologics and Office of Regulatory Affairs, *"Guidance on Sterile Drug Products Produced by Aseptic Processing."* F.D.A., Rockville, MD. 1987.

4. United States Pharmacopeial Convention, Inc., Sterile Drug Products for Home Use, <1206>. USP 24:2130-2143. 2000.

5. Peters, G. F., Laminar Airflow Equipment: Engineering Control of Aseptic Processing. In: *The Encyclopedia of Pharmaceutical Technology,* 1st Ed. 8:317-359 (J. Swarbrick and J. Boylan, Eds.), Marcel Dekker, Inc., NY. 1993.

6. National Sanitation Foundation, Advisory Committee for Biohazard Cabinetry. *NSF Standard No. 49,* Ann Arbor, MI. 1995.

7. ASHP technical assistance bulletin on handling cytotoxic and hazardous drugs. Am. J. Hosp. Pharm. 47:1033-49. 1990.

8. Bryan, D. and Marback, R. C., *Laminar-airflow equipment certification: What the pharmacist needs to know.* Am J. Hosp. Pharm., 41:1343-1349. 1984.

9. ASHP technical assistance bulletin on quality assurance for pharmacy-prepared sterile products. Am. J. Hosp. Pharm. 50:2386-2398. 1993.

10. Institute of Environmental Science and Technology. Federal Standard 209E. Airborne Particulate Cleanliness Classes in Cleanrooms and Clean zones. 1992.

11. Remington's Pharmaceutical Sciences, 17th Ed. p. 786. Mack Publishing. Easton, PA. 1985.

12. Welker, R., *Controlling particle transfer caused by cleanroom gloves.* Microcontamination. 17(8):61-65, 1999.

13. Galalowitsh, S., *Technique may be the culprit behind Class II BSC contamination.* Cleanrooms. 13(11): 1, 4, 45. 1999.

14. OSHA, *Work Practice Guidelines for Personnel Dealing with Cytotoxic (Antineoplastic) Drugs.* Instr. Pub. 8.1.1, U.S. Dept. Labor, Washington D.C. 1986.

15. Reifman, N., *"Math Master" Pharmaceutical Calculations,* 2nd Ed. Evergreen, CO. Ark Pharmaceutical Consultants, Inc. 2001. 1-800-798-3247.

INDEX

A

Absorption, natural routes i,2
Additives
    Injecting into Bags and Bottles 57
    Injecting Additives into a Bottle 60
    Injecting into a Bottle with Vent Tube 60
    Injecting into a Plastic Bag 58
    Needle-less Systems 61
Administration and Drip Rates 83
Alcohol 30, 34-35
Disinfection 34
Allergens 4
Ampules 51-54
    Filling Syringe 53
    Opening 52
Anterooms 10, 21, 32
Arrangement of Materials
    in a BSC 41
    in an HFCB 39
    in a VFCB 40
Assessments, written and practical viii
Aseptic processing 1, 2
Aseptic Technique 6, 7, 64
Aseptic Manipulations 30
Automated Compounders 62-64

B

Backwash Contamination 14
Bags With End-Type Additive Ports 59
Bags With "Belly Port" 59
Barrier Controls 6, 23
Bevel, Needle 30
Biological Safety Cabinet (BSC) 10

BSC (Biological Safety Cabinet)
    Airflow Patterns 16, 17
    Arrangement of Materials 41-42
    Classification, BSC 15-16
    Cleaning 35-37
    Limitations 18-19
    Operation, 24-hour 19
    Performance Testing 19
    Types 15-16
Buffer Zone 19-20

C

Calculations, Pharmaceutical 71
Calibration 32, 62-64
Changing Needles 46
Compounding Devices, Automated 62
    One-Solution Pumps 63
    Multiple-Solution Pumps 63-64
Compounding Tools
    Other 64-66
    Selection 42-45
Contaminant 1
Conversion,
    Equivalent Weights 86
    Factor 75
    Units of Measure 74-77
Core 30
Coring 47
Cross-Stream Contamination 14,15
Cross-contamination 1, 4, 42
Critical Site 11, 13, 40, 41, 45, 47, 64, 65

D

Deadly Decimal Point 78-79, 81, 85
Definitions, explained vii
Disinfectant 30, 34
Dispensing Pins 44, 54-56
Dosage and Dilution Calculations 85-90
Downstream Contamination 14

V

Vacuum, in bottles 60, 61
Validation 2
     and monitoring 5
Variable 2, 4-5
Vertical Flow Clean Bench (VFCB) 11
     Arrangement of Materials 40
     Cleaning 35
Vials, Reconstituting 50-51, 57
Volume-to-Volume Percentage
     Expressions 79

W

Water Manometer 20
Weight-to-Weight Percentage
     Expressions 79
Weight-to-Volume Percentage
     Expressions 79

NOTES: